working on MySelf, bY mYSELF, for Myself

MY SELF LOVE
JOURNAL & ACTIVITY BOOK

Qur'an Shakir

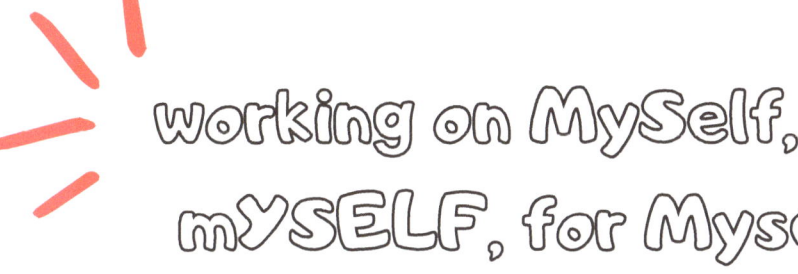

ISBN: 979-8-9896332-4-1
Published by Shakir Enterprises
BUBI - Building Us Beyond Imagination Publishing
October 2024
Atlanta, Georgia
United States of America, USA

Copyrighted 2024

All rights reserved. No part of this book may be reproduced or used in any manner without the prior written permission of the copyright owner, except for the use of brief quotations in a book review.

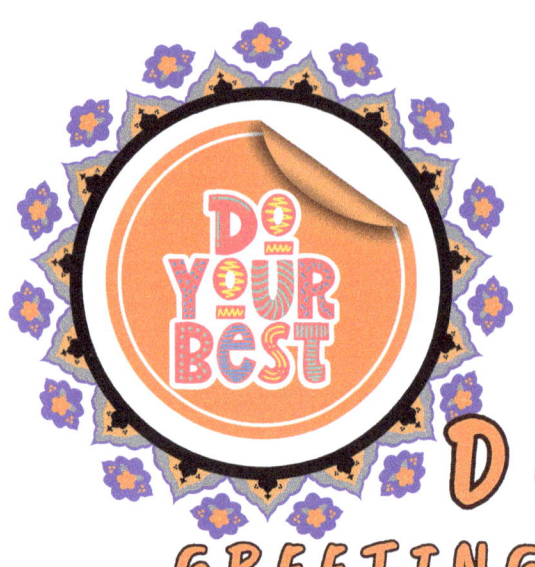
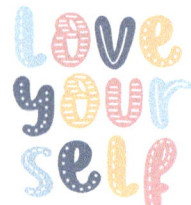

DEDICATION

GREETINGS!

I am so excited that YOU ARE HERE sharing this book, these pages, this time. I am excited because I believe it is very important when you want to be your best self that you take time to speak with yourself, be with yourself, release and embrace yourself.

I share these tools, this love offering, to all of the young people that sometimes feel sad, lonely, confused, hurt, or down. You are seen. You are heard. You are loved. You are valued. You are needed.

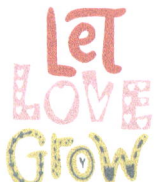

Beloved, let your "best self" naturally evolve and make a home inside of you. One of the best ways to do that is to sometimes sit alone with your thoughts. As one sits with their thoughts, writing those thoughts down, even simply doodling, helps with getting to know yourself better and with planning your future, your life, directing and managing your own joy. Know also the value of community and bringing your great energy and joy into healthy space. That identification begins with you.

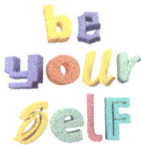

Feel free to color, draw, fill in wherever your heart moves your hands and heart to do so. This is your book. Use it to express, release, discover, find joy!

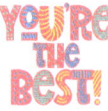

Madame Q

celebratingsacredconnections@gmail.com

ABOUT THIS ACTIVITY & WORKBOOK

Use this book and these activities to become regular routines in your life. When you do, you can develop mindfulness, emotional awareness, and positive habits in an engaging and supportive way.

Some things to do in this book:

INCORPORATE MINDFULNESS GAMES INTO DAILY ROUTINE
Choose one of the mindfulness games from the book to develop focus and present-moment awareness in a fun and engaging way.

SOLVE THE PUZZLES
Develop your problem-solving skills while fostering a mindful approach to challenges by completing a puzzle or maze from this book at the end of he day, as a way to wind down your day

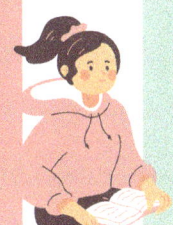

SET AND TRACK GOALS
Use the goal-setting activities and calendars of the book to set personal goals like reading a certain number of books or learning a new skill. Setting and tracking goals will help you learn about planning, perseverance, and celebrating small achievements.

IMPLEMENT FOOD TRACKING AND HEALTHY EATING
Use the food tracking pages to monitor eating habits. record what you eat and explore which food choices make you feel good.

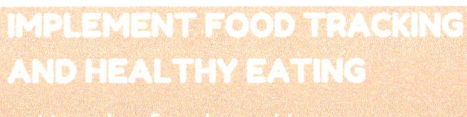

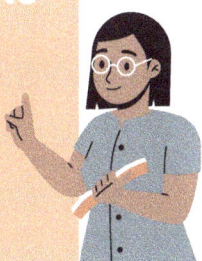

CREATE A MINDFULNESS ROUTINE
Develop a daily or weekly mindfulness routine incorporating activities from the book. For example, start with a short mindfulness exercise, followed by a puzzle, and end with a gratitude journal entry.

EXPLORE JOURNAL PROMPTS ON GRATITUDE AND POSITIVITY
Each day or week, take time to respond to a journal prompt which are about great topics like gratitude, smiling, and picking good friends. You might write about three things you are grateful for or describe a time when you made a new friend. All of this can help you have a positive mindset and enhance emotional intelligence.

CUSTOMIZE ACTIVITIES BASED ON INTERESTS
This book includes variety of activities. Try different ones, not just what you like. Try drawing, creating art, writing about gratitude, breathing and doing the mindfulness practices, and thinking deeply about art. It is all beneficial in growing you into a young person who is able to balance emotions and participate in things you like as well as unfamiliar things.

SHARE WHAT YOU HAVE LEARNED
Celebrate the things you learn through this book with your family and friends. You can share during family meals or special family time. Doing this can strengthen family bonds and provide a supportive environment for practicing mindfulness.

HAVE FUN!
No matter what you do, please enjoy every page of this book and the great activities.

A MOMENT TO PAUSE, BREATHE, AND FEEL CALM AGAIN

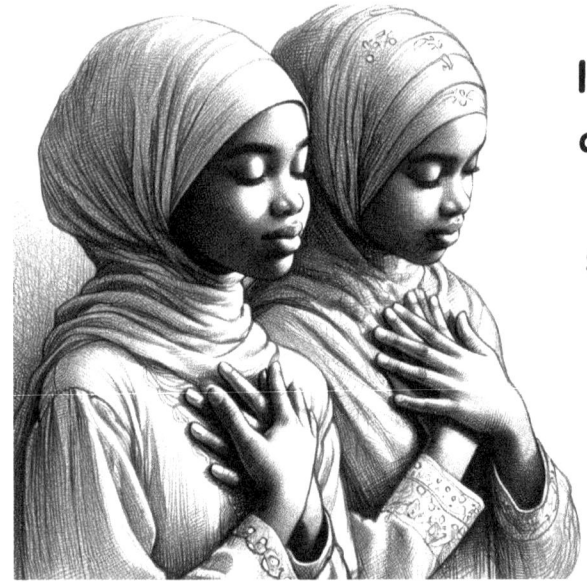

Imagine that your mind is like a busy room, filled with a lot of thoughts and feelings— some good, but others that can make you feel worried, scared, or even mad.

When these feelings start to feel too big, like a balloon that's about to pop, prayer can be like a gentle needle that slowly helps you release and let the air out.

Prayer is a special way to talk to The Almighty. When you feel anxious, afraid, or upset, praying can help you feel like you're not alone.

It's like having a trusted friend or guide who listens to you and cares about what you're going through.

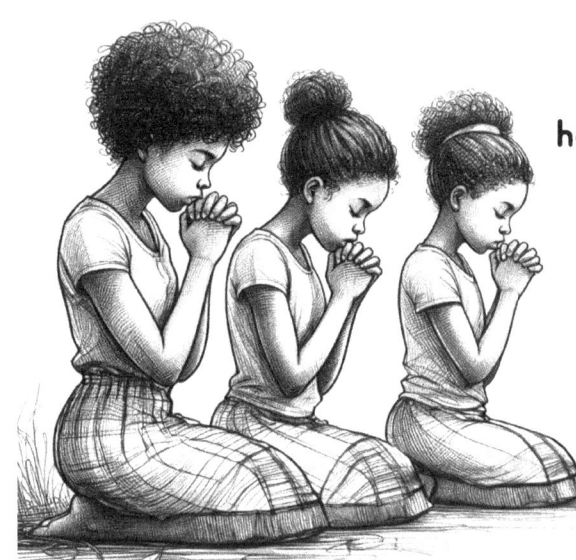

You can tell The Creator how you feel, and it helps you to let go of those heavy emotions.

When you pray, it's like taking all that big, scary energy and turning it into something softer and calmer inside of you.

Just like when you hug someone you love and feel comforted, prayer can bring peace to your heart and mind.

It reminds you that you are safe, loved, and that things will be okay, even when they seem hard.

ONE MORE THING ABOUT PRAYER:

PRAY! THEN ACT!

Imagine you're trying to grow a plant. If you just ask for the plant to grow but never water it, it won't work, right? You need to both care for it and ask for help. That's the same with prayer! Prayer is like asking The Almighty for help, but our actions are like watering the plant. You can't just pray and do nothing—you need to put in the effort too.

For example, if you pray to do well in school, but you don't study or try your best, the prayer alone won't help. The Almighty loves it when we pray and work hard. Prayer gives us strength, and our actions show we're really trying. It's like saying, "I trust you, The Almighty, and I'm doing my part too!" When we combine prayer with good actions, amazing things can happen.

It's a moment to pause, breathe, and feel calm again.

WAYS TO PRAY

Talking to The Almighty

You can pray by simply talking to The Almighty in your own words, just like you talk to a friend or family member. You can tell The Almighty how you feel, ask for help, or say thank you.

Reciting Prayers

Some people use special words from their faith. For example, Muslims say prayers from the Qur'an, like "Surah Al-Fatiha" or "Ayatul-Qursi," which ask The Almighty for protection and guidance.

Silent Prayer

You can pray in your heart without speaking out loud. Just close your eyes and think your prayer to The Almighty.

Breathing and Calming

You can combine prayer with breathing slowly. As you breathe in, ask The Almighty to give you peace, and as you breathe out, let go of your worry.

If you want to talk to The Almighty, pray!

If you want The Almighty to talk to you, meditate!

Write About It

Prophets' Prayers for Anxiety Relief:
How Different Prophets Talked to The Almighty When Feeling Anxious or Scared

Prophet Moses (Musa) (peace be upon him)

When Prophet Moses was asked by The Almighty to speak to Pharaoh, he felt nervous and anxious because Pharaoh was a powerful king. So Moses prayed, asking The Almighty for help:

"O my Lord! Open for me my chest (relieve my mind), and ease my task for me." (Qur'an 20:25-26)
Moses asked for calmness and confidence to do the difficult task.

Prophet Jonah (Yunus) (peace be upon him)

Prophet Jonah felt scared and alone when he was inside the belly of a big fish. In that dark moment, he prayed to The Almighty for help, saying:

"There is no god but You, Glory be to You! Truly, I have been of the wrongdoers." (Qur'an 21:87).
His prayer was one of asking for forgiveness and help from The Almighty, and The Almighty saved him.

Prophet Muhammed (peace be upon him)

When Prophet Muhammed felt afraid during difficult times, he would often pray. One of his prayers when he felt anxious or worried was:

**"O My Lord, I seek refuge in You from worry and grief, from weakness and laziness, from cowardice and miserliness, from being overwhelmed by debt and the oppression of humankind."**

Prophet Jesus (Isa) (peace be upon him)

When Prophet Jesus met people who were unkind to him, he prayed for them, asking The Almighty to forgive them. Jesus prayed: **"Our Father in heaven, hallowed be Your name. Your kingdom come, Your will be done, on earth as it is in heaven. Give us this day our daily bread, and forgive us our debts, as we forgive our debtors."** (Bible, Matthew 6:9-13)

WHAT IS MINDFULNESS?

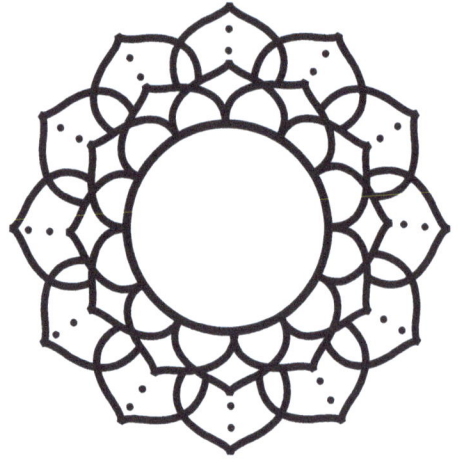

Mindfulness is a practice of gently focusing your awareness on the present moment and being fully engaged with whatever you're doing at the moment — free from distraction or judgment.

BEING MINDFUL...

- improves brain activity and creativity
- boosts mood and self-esteem
- reduces stress, worries, and regrets
- improves quality of sleep
- encourages positive behavior
- improves decision making ability
- helps develop stronger relationships

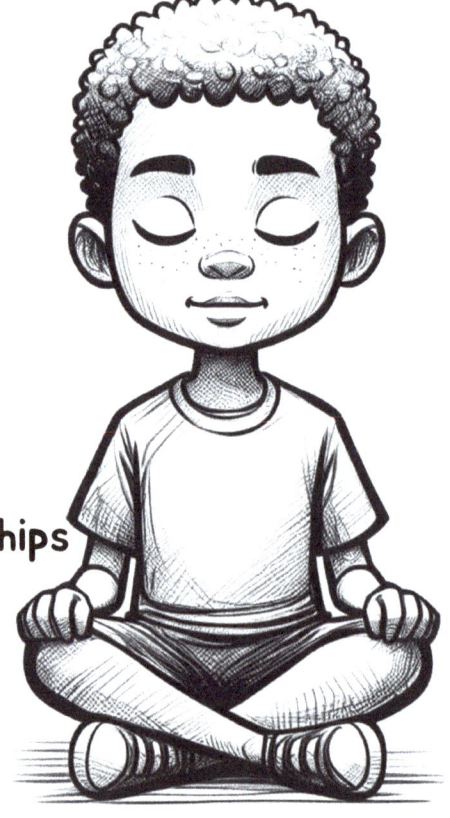

MINDFULNESS IS A SUPERPOWER.

MINDFULNESS ACTIVITY

Practice paying attention to your breath to calm your body. Take full breaths by tracing the lines with your finger as you breathe in and out.

- INHALE FOR THREE
- HOLD FOR TWO
- EXHALE FOR THREE

What emotions came up in your body and mind during this activity? Did your mind wander? What did you think about?

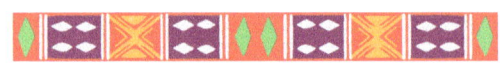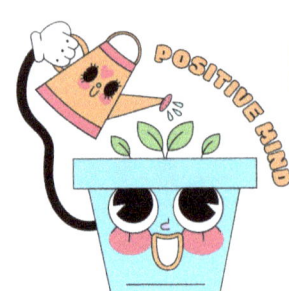

7 QUALITIES LOVED by THE DIVINE ONE......

TAWBAH (Repentance)
"For Allah Loves those who turn to Him Constantly (in repentance)" (Surat Al-Baqarah 2:222)

TAQWA (Piety)
"For Allah Loves the righteous (the pious)" (Surat Al-Tawabah 9:4)

IHSAN (Goodness and Perfection)
"For Allah Loves those who do good" (Surah Al Imran 3:134)

TAHARAH (Purification)
Allah Loves those who keep themselves pure and clean " (Surah Al-Baqarah 2:222)

ADL (Justice)
For Allah Loves those who judge in equity." (Surah Al Maidah 5:42)

SABR (Patience)
And Allah Loves those who are firm and steadfast (As-Sabinn) (the patient) (Surah Al Imran 3:146).

TAWWAKAL (Trust)
For Allah Loves those who put their trust (in Him) Surah Al Imran 3:159)

ALL ABOUT ME

MY NAME IS BEAUTIFULLY MADE

Write your full name.

I AM SPECIAL IN MY OWN WAY

Draw your self-portrait.

MY FAMILY LOVES ME

Draw and label your family portrait.

EATING GIVES ME ENERGY

Draw or write about your favourite foods.

PLAYING HELPS ME TO LEARN

Draw or write about your favourite activities.

ME

WHAT I AM FEELING IS

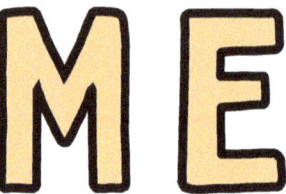

MY NAME MEANS

Find out the meaning of your name. Who named you? Why did they give you your name?

Are you named after someone? Who? Would you like to also write about that person?

TRY GROUNDING

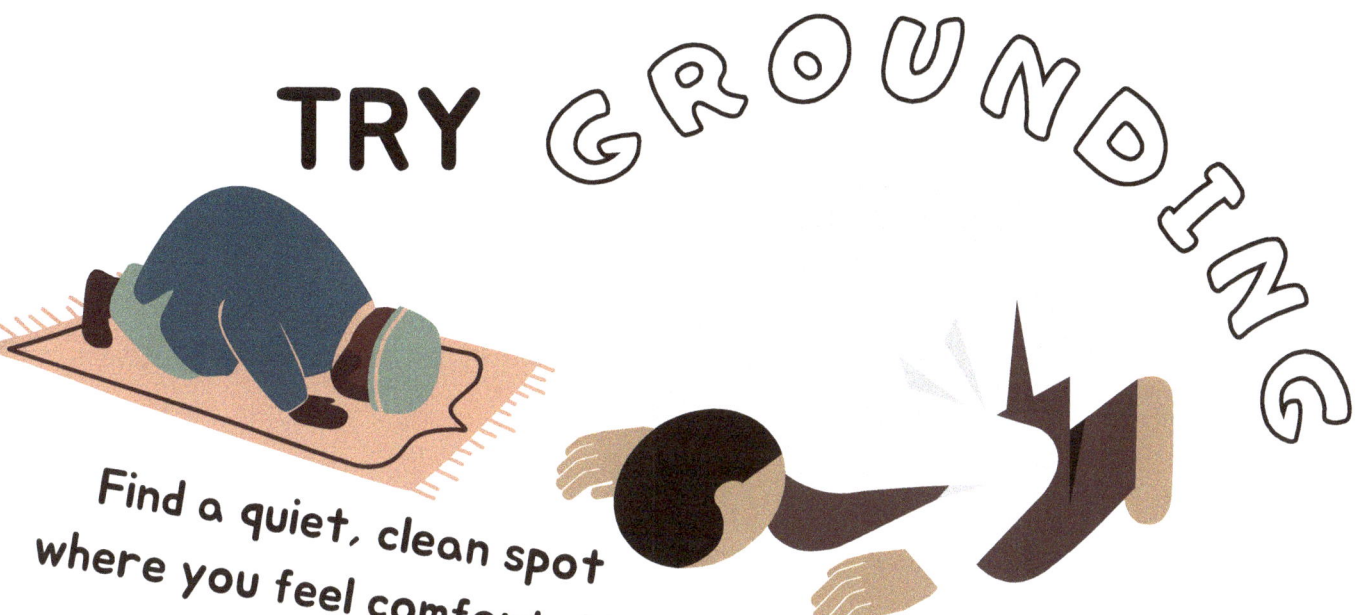

Find a quiet, clean spot where you feel comfortable.

Kneel down, then bend forward, gently lowering your head until your forehead touches the ground.

Relax your body and take slow, deep breaths.

Feel the ground beneath you and imagine you're letting all your worries go into the earth.

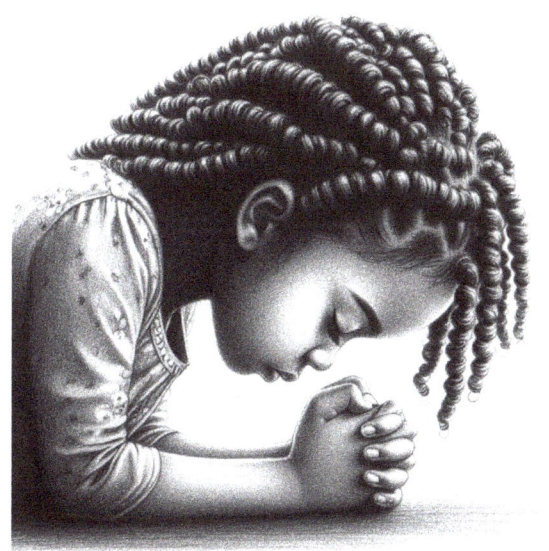

Stay like that for a moment, breathing slowly, then sit up when you feel ready.

Grounding with the Earth

Take a moment to think about a time when you felt peaceful and calm. Now imagine yourself pressing your forehead or feet against the ground, like you're giving the earth a big hug.

1. How does it feel to connect with the earth?

2. What do you imagine happens inside your body when you do this?

3. How does grounding help you let go of any worries or stress?

Write about a time when you felt anxious or upset. How might grounding, like placing your forehead on the ground, help you feel better?

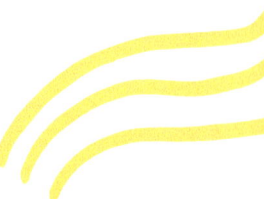

WHY I matter

NOTES TO SELF

TUNING IN WITH YOUR FIVE SENSES

Use the 54321 grounding exercise to help you focus on the present moment and tune in to what is happening around you.

5 THINGS I SEE

4 THINGS I FEEL

3 THINGS I HEAR

2 THINGS I SMELL

1 THING I TASTE

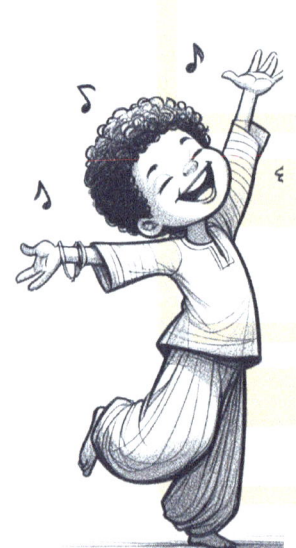
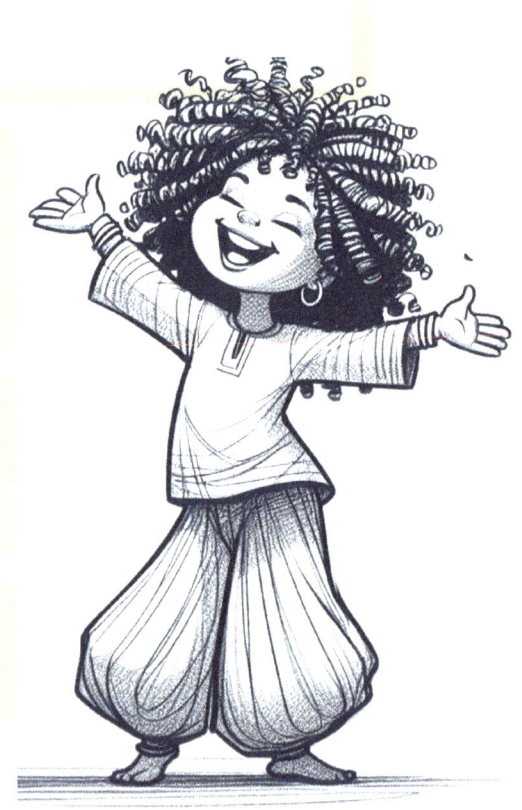

YOUR THOUGHTS
DAILY JOURNAL

DATES :   MOOD :

....

....

....

....

....

....

....

GOAL   ## TO DO LIST

-
-
-
-
-
-
-

Angry	Happy	Sad
Nervous	Excited	Calm
_____	_____	_____

PUSH THROUGH

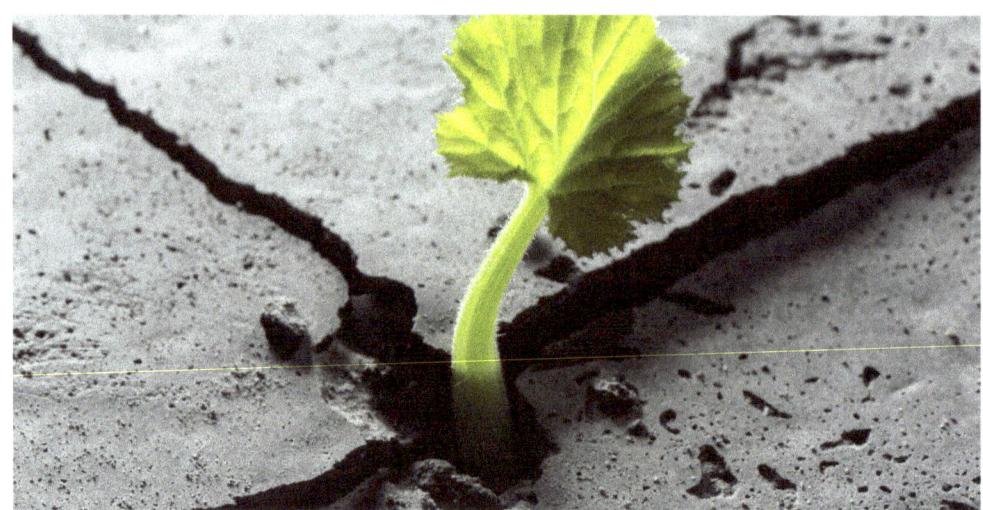

YOUR THOUGHTS:

What does it mean to 'push through'? What does it take to 'push through'? What do you think you need in order to 'push through'?

....

....

....

....

....

....

....

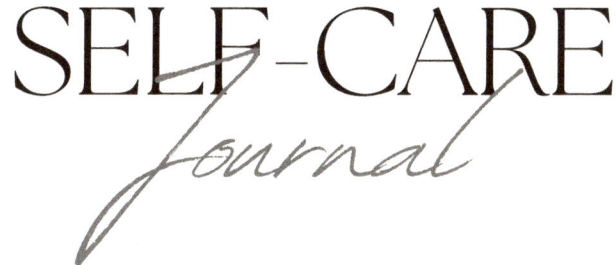

DATE: /   /

● ● ● ● ● ● ●
S M T W T F S

TODAY I'M GRATEFUL FOR:

1. ....

2. ....

3. ....

WATER INTAKE

💧 💧 💧 💧 💧 💧 💧 💧
1 2 3 4 5 6 7 8   (Glass)

MOOD

😠   😟   😢   🙂   😂
ANGRY   TIRED   SAD   HAPPY   EXCITED

TODAY'S AFFIRMATION

....

....

....

....

NOTES/REMINDER:

....

....

....

FOR TOMORROW

....

....

....

THERMOMETER

Taking your emotional temperature throughout the day helps you listen to your body's needs, recognize triggers, and increase awareness of your emotions, allowing you to implement strategies before negative feelings escalate and improve your relationships with yourself and others.

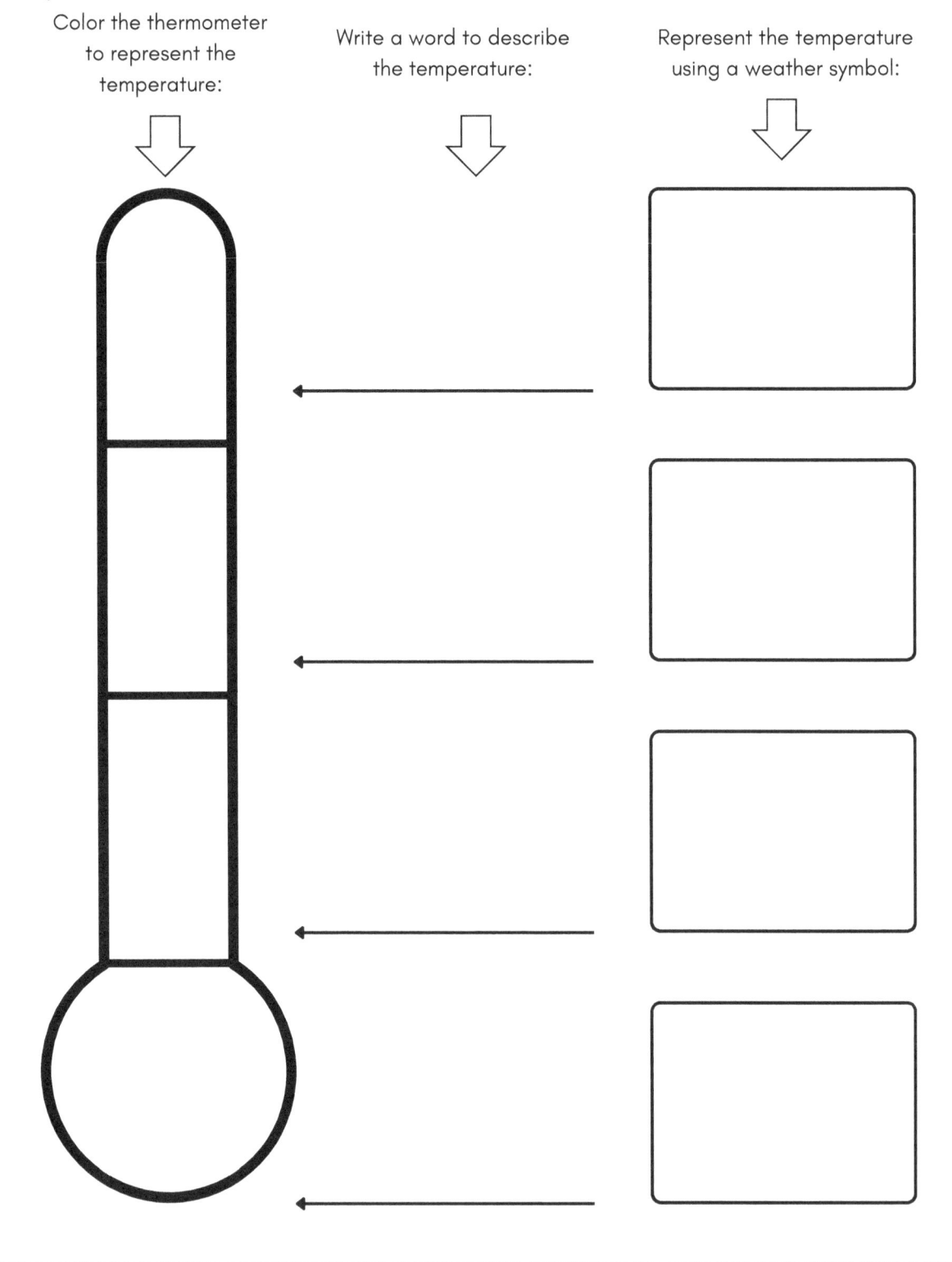

FIVE SENSES HUNT

Search your home or space for different objects, draw them on the chart and then mark if you can hear, see, touch, smell or taste them

Can you hear, see, touch, smell or taste it?	👂	👁	✋	👃	👅
1					
2					
3					
4					
5					
6					

FEELINGS

Feelings can be complicated. Sometimes it's hard to say how we are feeling. We can always start by identifying if we feel good, or bad.

FEELING GOOD?

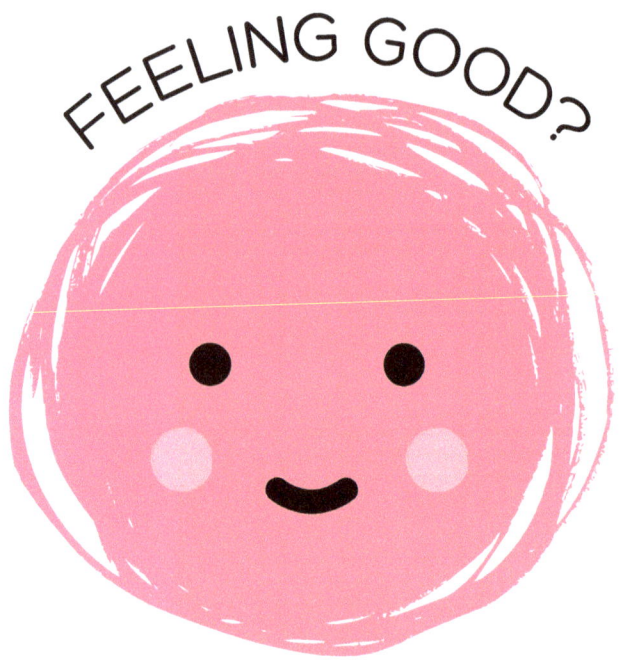

FEELING BAD?

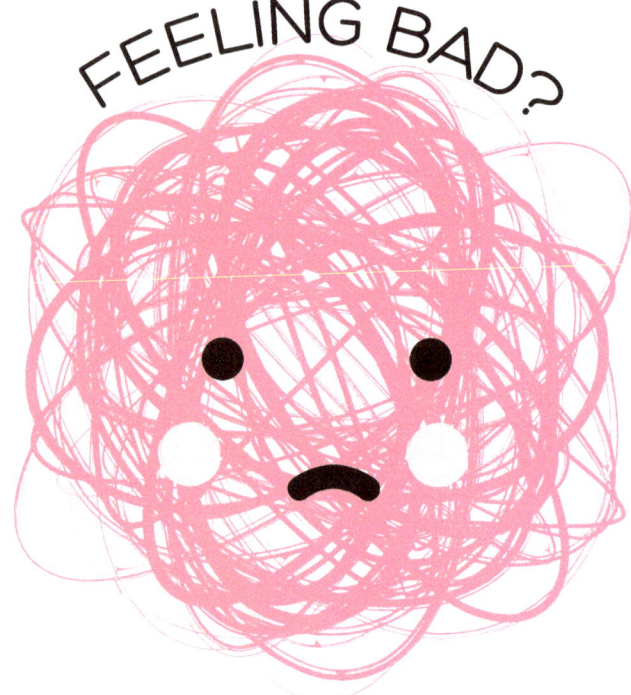

When you feel good, you might also say, I feel …

- happy
- joyful
- confident
- proud
- calm
- excited

When you feel bad, you might also say, I feel …

- sad
- angry
- frustrated
- scared
- worried
- mad

ALL OUR FEELINGS ARE OKAY!

MY THOUGHTS

Write or draw any thoughts that keep coming up.

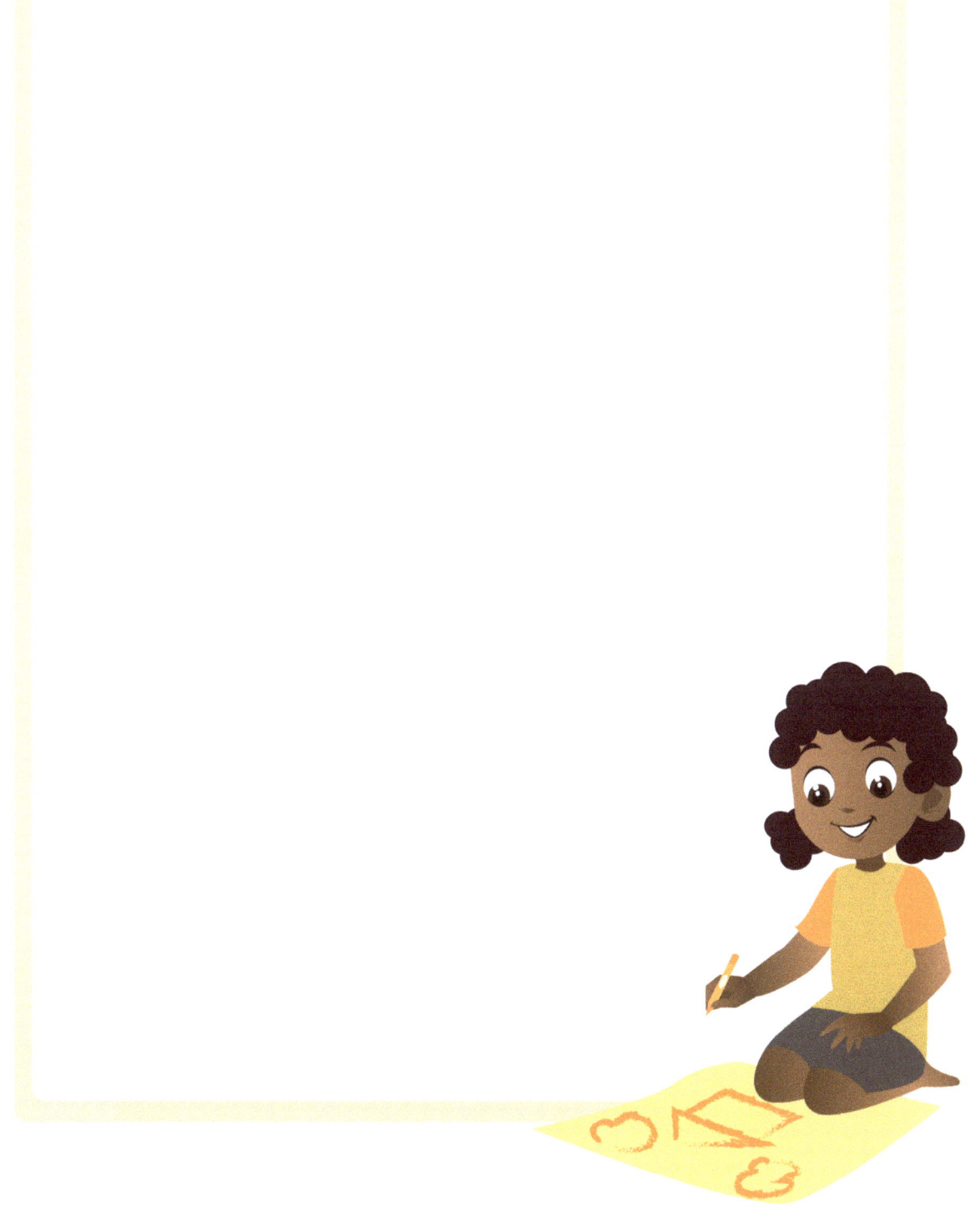

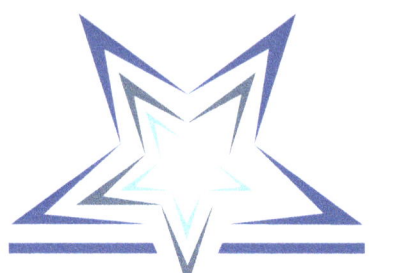

WEEKLY PLANNER

WHAT DO YOU WANT TO ACCOMPLISH THIS WEEK? WORK ON YOUR PASSIONS DAILY. WHAT WILL YOU DO EACH DAY? WRITE IT DOWN HERE.

MONDAY

TUESDAY

WEDNESDAY

THURSDAY

FRIDAY

SATURDAY

NOTES AND IDEA

SMART GOALS

Setting realistic and achievable outcomes. Think about 1-3 goals you want to achieve. Make the goals SMART.

My goal is:

S — SPECIFIC
What do I want to happen?

M — MEASUREABLE
How will I know when I have achieved my goal?

A — ATTAINABLE
Is the goal realistic and how will I accomplish it?

R — RELEVANT
Why is my goal important to me?

T — TIMELY
What is my deadline for this goal?

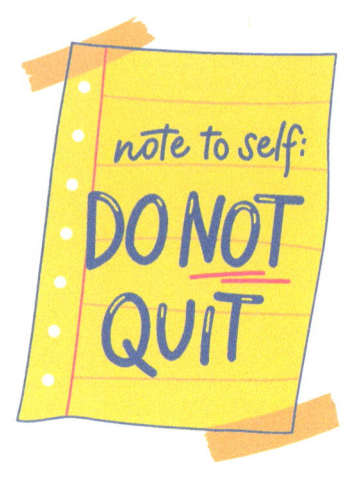
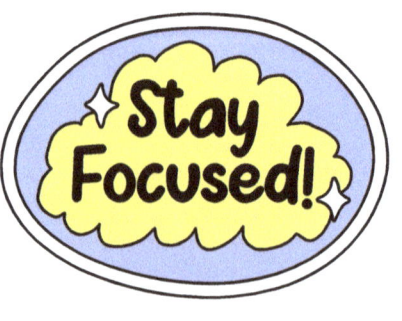

THE Healing POWER OF A HUG

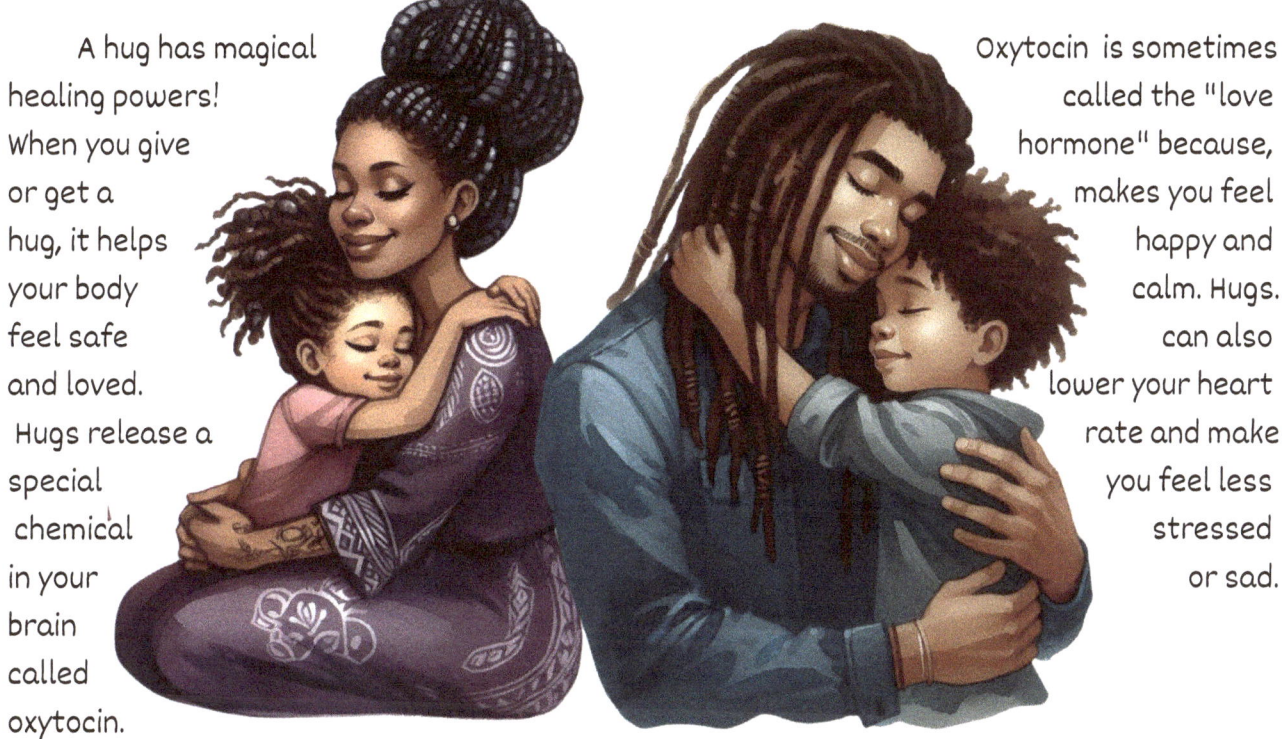

A hug has magical healing powers! When you give or get a hug, it helps your body feel safe and loved. Hugs release a special chemical in your brain called oxytocin.

Oxytocin is sometimes called the "love hormone" because, makes you feel happy and calm. Hugs can also lower your heart rate and make you feel less stressed or sad.

How to Hug:
A healthy, healing hug should last at least 20 seconds. That might feel like a long time, but that's when your body starts to feel calm and releases those feel-good chemicals and lowers the heart rate. It's like giving yourself and the person you're hugging a little moment of love and care!

Try a Heart-to-Heart Hug:
A heart-to-heart hug is when you hug someone so that your hearts are close to each other (lean a little to the left). This kind of hug feels extra warm and comforting because it's like your hearts are talking to each other!

A hug of 10 seconds boosts the immune system, eases sadness, and makes you feel less tired.

So, next time you give someone a hug, remember—take a deep breath, hold it for a while, and let your hearts connect. It's one of the easiest ways to feel better!

All About Me

Name

Age **Birthday**

Address

My Hobbies

My Favorite ...

Color: ....

Food: ....

Pet: ....

Music: ....

Movie: ....

Season: ....

Place: ....

Sports: ....

Subject: ....

Scriptural verse: ....

Fun Facts About Me

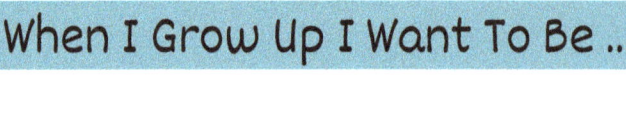
When I Grow Up I Want To Be ...

Name: _____   Date: _____

Today's REFLECTION

Today is:

How I feel about today:

☹ 😐 😶 🙂 😃

My act of kindness:

Reason for my rating
_____
_____
_____
_____
_____
_____

Something new I learned today:
_____
_____
_____

OH WORRY! DEAR WORRY!

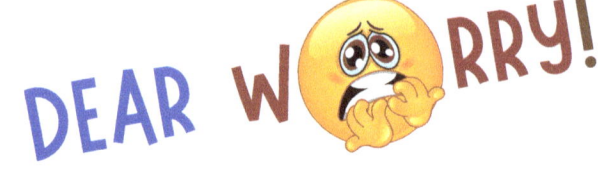

Oh, worry, dear worry, it visits us all,
It can feel like a storm or a voice in the hall.
It sneaks in your head, when you least expect,
And suddenly things seem much worse than they get!

But why do we worry? Why all the fuss?
It's because we want safety, for things to be just.

We wonder, "What if?" and, "What could go wrong?"
But sometimes, dear child, that worry's too strong.

You see, worry's a thought that tries to protect,
But sometimes it grows, and it has an effect.

It makes your heart race, and your mind starts to spin,
But don't worry! There's ways you can help from within!

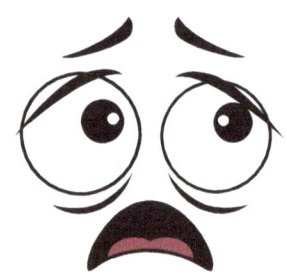

Take a deep breath, in and out, nice and slow,
And imagine a place where the calm breezes blow.
Talk to someone, share your thoughts if you can,
A friend or a grown-up will lend you a hand.

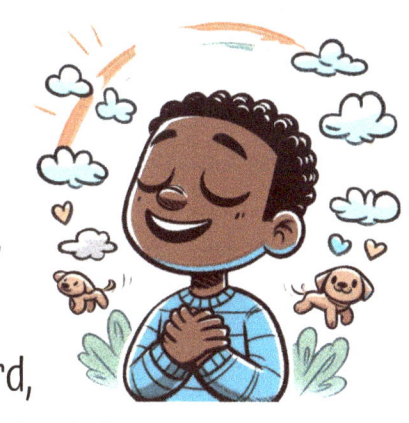

"Close your eyes,
        count to ten,
                find a happy space,
Picture puppies or rainbows, a warm, cozy place!
      Sometimes a worry just needs to be heard,
          Once it's out of your mind, it feels less absurd.

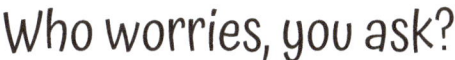

        Who worries, you ask?
          Oh, all people do!
    Moms, dads, and teachers—yep, them too!
     Even big giants and folks who are wise,
   Sometimes have worries that cloud up their skies.

But here's something special I'll share just with you:
You're stronger than worries, it's perfectly true.

You push through the fear,
with courage and cheer,
And soon all those worries will start to clear!

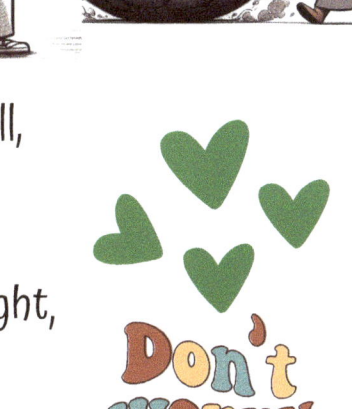

So when worry comes knocking, don't fret or feel small,
You can rise up above it, you'll handle it all!

With deep breaths and love, and thoughts that are bright,
You'll push through the worry and be all right.

MY W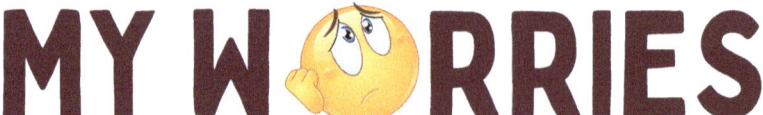RRIES

Write down all of your worries that keep coming up.

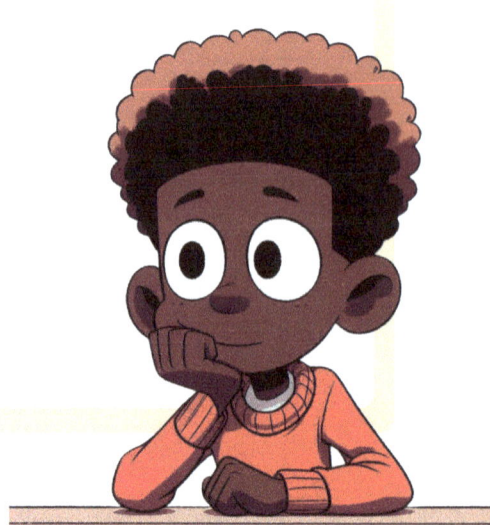

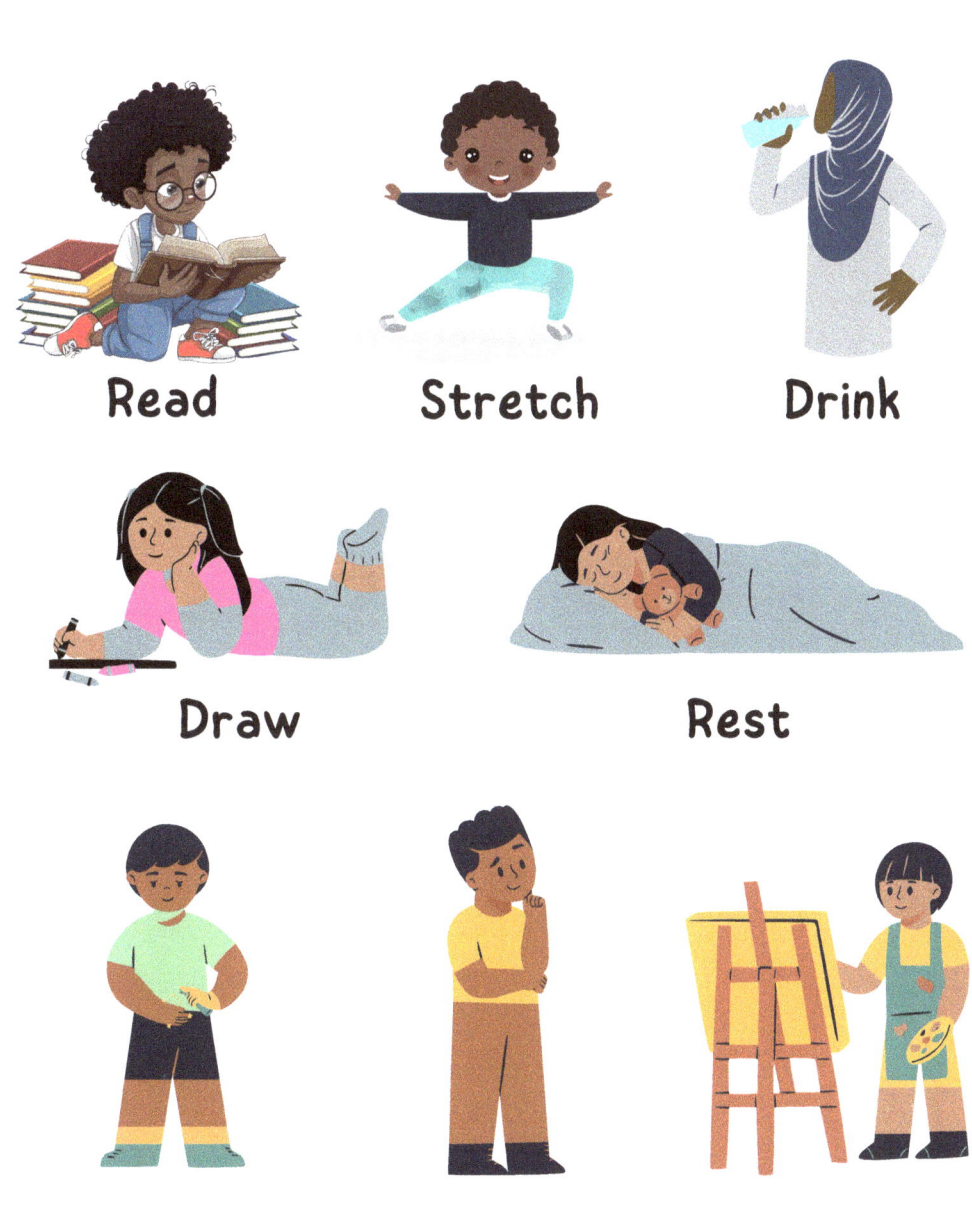

WHAT CAN HELP...

Draw, write or describe what can help you when you are feeling each of these emotions.

When I feel stressed...

When I need a break...

When I feel hurt...

When I feel angry...

When I feel worried...

COPING TOOLS
WHAT HELPS ME

- ☐ Take slow, mindful breaths
- ☐ Drink a warm cup of water
- ☐ Rest and take a break
- ☐ Stretch
- ☐ Journal or write a letter
- ☐ Listen to your favorite music
- ☐ Talk to someone you trust
- ☐ Get a hug
- ☐ Cuddle or play with your pet
- ☐ Use positive affirmations
- ☐ Use a stress ball
- ☐ Blow bubbles
- ☐ Make an artwork
- ☐ Hug or climb a tree
- ☐ Read a book or magazine
- ☐ Take a shower or bath

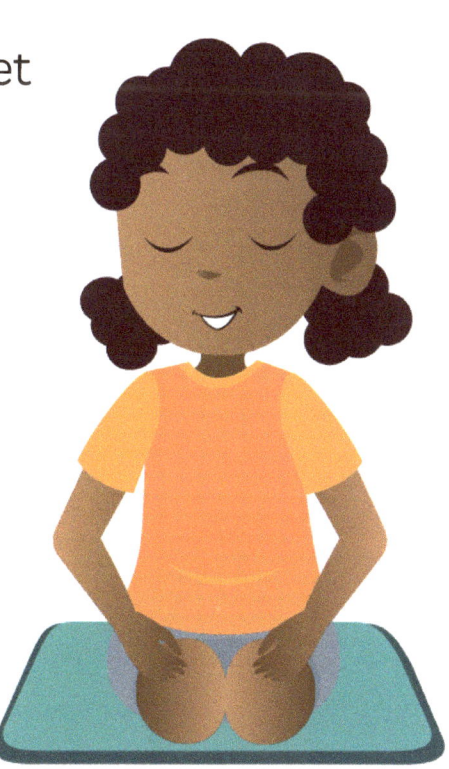

Name: _____ Date: _____

IDENTIFYING TRIGGERS

Which of the following makes you feel angry?

- ☐ Someone says you did something wrong.
- ☐ Someone belittles you.
- ☐ You want something you cannot have.
- ☐ Someone shouts at you.
- ☐ You are told you can't do something right.
- ☐ Someone doesn't agree with you.
- ☐ You are unable to finish your task.
- ☐ You are feeling left out.
- ☐ There's too many people.
- ☐ There's too much noise.
- ☐ Someone is disturbing you.
- ☐ There's too much homework.
- ☐ There's too much housework.
- ☐ Someone criticizes you.
- ☐ Someone hurts you.
- ☐ Someone threatens you.
- ☐ Someone laughs at you.

Make the RIGHT MOVE

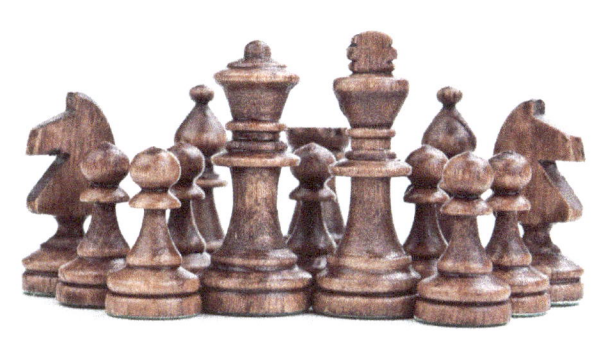

Life is about making the right decisions, the right moves. When you think about the things you will do, think also about the outcomes of the decision.

Share a decision you made that was the right decision. Explain.

Share a decision you made that was not the best decision. Explain. What lessons did you learn? What would you do differently?

WEEKLY PLANNER

WHAT DO YOU WANT TO ACCOMPLISH THIS WEEK? WORK ON YOUR PASSIONS DAILY. WHAT WILL YOU DO EACH DAY? WRITE IT DOWN HERE.

MONDAY

TUESDAY

WEDNESDAY

THURSDAY

FRIDAY

SATURDAY

NOTES AND IDEA

....

....

....

....

ALL ABOUT ME!

My name is _____

I am _____ years old.

I am from _____

I am excited about _____
_____
_____

My superpowers

During my free time, I like to:

My Favorite Book is:

My Favorite Foods are:

Healthy or Unhealthy?

Identify each food item and mark the correct option.

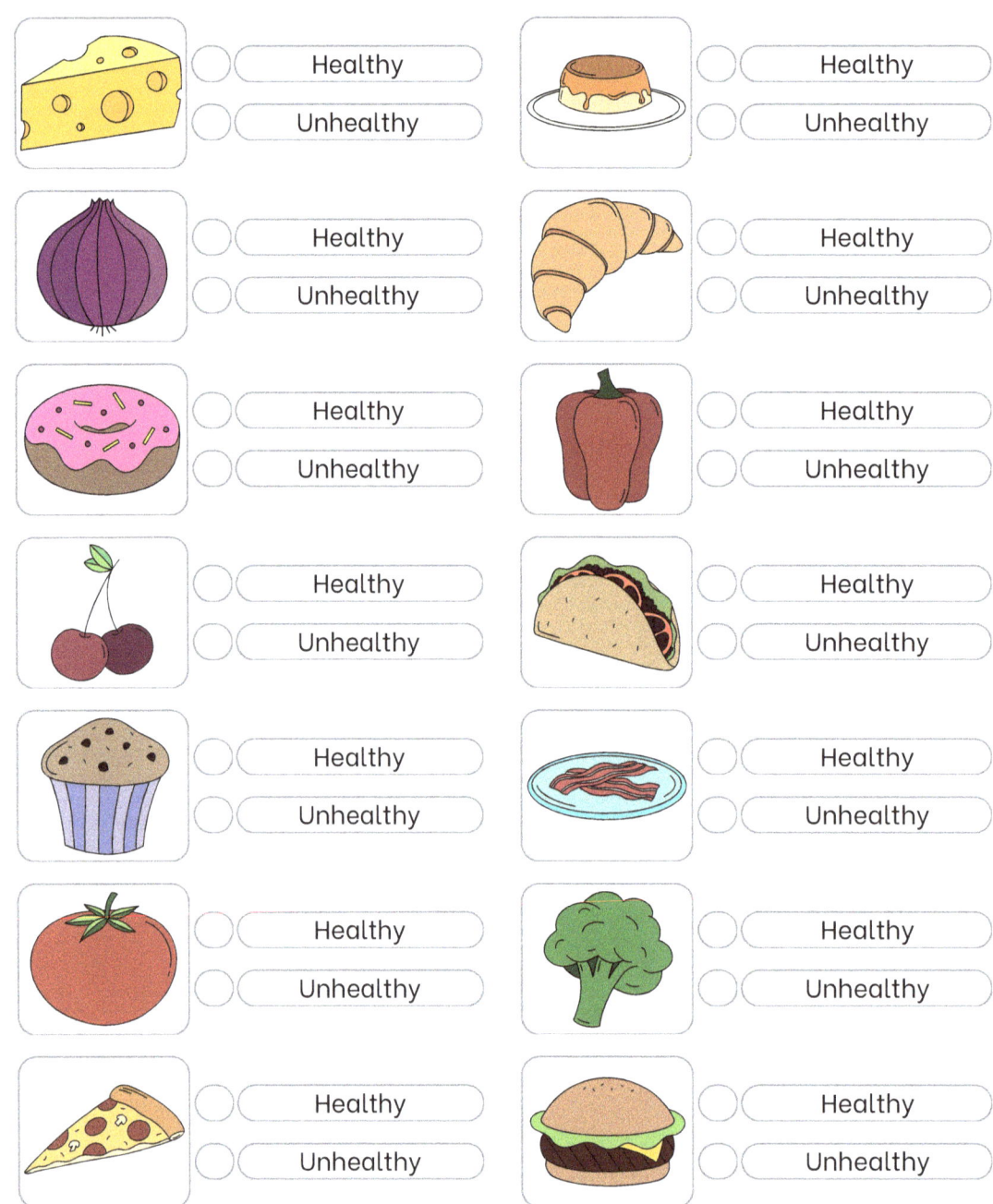

EAT WELL

Write about the foods you put in your body this week. How much of what you ate was good for your growth and health? Explain.

How much of the foods you ate were not the best for your growth and health? Why do you think you chose to eat that food?

DAILY REFLECTION

Date: _____

Three moments you'd like to remember:

One thing that inspired you:

One thing that surprised you:

One person who made you smile:

One thing you accomplished:

Art Comparison

Use the spaces below to compare the two different works of art.

Artwork 1
Title: Barber Shop
Artist: Jacob Lawrence
Year Made: 1946

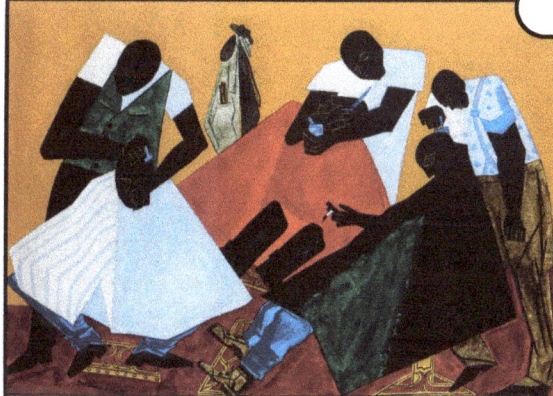

Similarities
What makes these two pieces of art similar?

Write your answer here.....

Differences
- What makes these two pieces of art different?

    Write your answer here.....

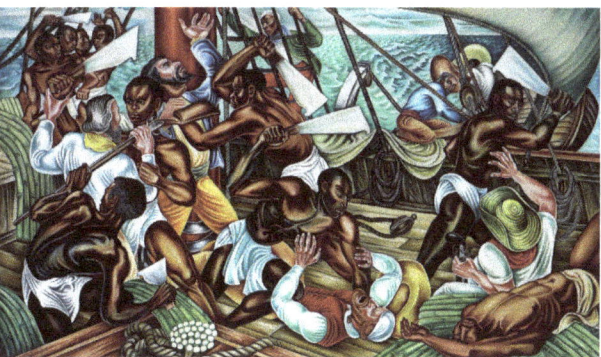

Artwork 2
Title: The Amistad Murals
Artist: Hale Aspacio Woodruff
Year Made: 1936

SELF REFLECTION

ROSE, THORN AND BUD

Rose means something positive that happened. Thorn is something you need help with, a challenge for you. Bud is a new idea or something to look forward to. Reflect in writing on your week's experience. Write about your rose, thorn, and bud.

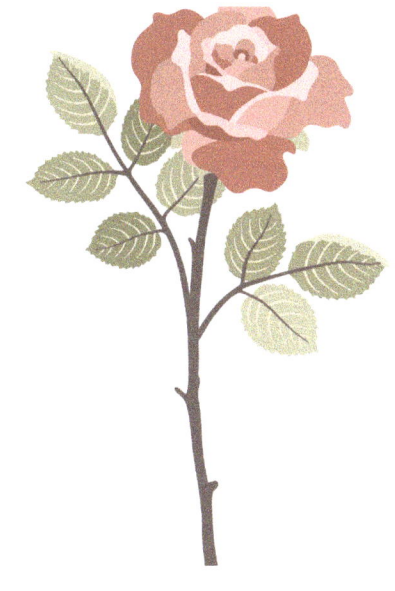

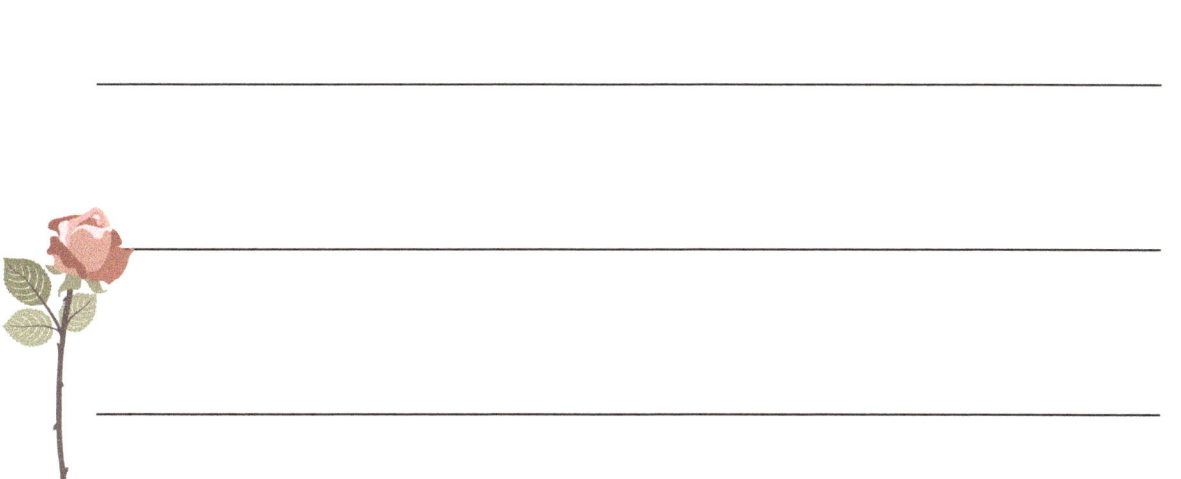

Writing Task Cards

Choose a card from the list and write about it.

What are your favorite things to do over the weekend?	Describe your family. (Pets are included.)
What is the best vacation you have ever taken?	What is your favorite part of the school day? Why?
What fictional character would you like to be? Why?	What is the best day of the week? Why?

WEEKLY PLANNER

WHAT DO YOU WANT TO ACCOMPLISH THIS WEEK? WORK ON YOUR PASSIONS DAILY. WHAT WILL YOU DO EACH DAY? WRITE IT DOWN HERE.

MONDAY

TUESDAY

WEDNESDAY

THURSDAY

FRIDAY

SATURDAY

NOTES AND IDEA

Name: _____   Date: _____

Today's REFLECTION

Today is:

How I feel about today:

☹ 😐 🙂 😊 😀

My act of kindness:

Reason for my rating

_____
_____
_____
_____
_____
_____

Something new I learned today:

_____
_____
_____

A Maze Game

Draw a line to help the child find their way to their friends.

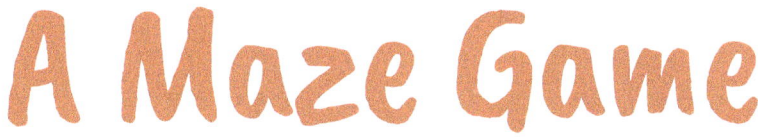

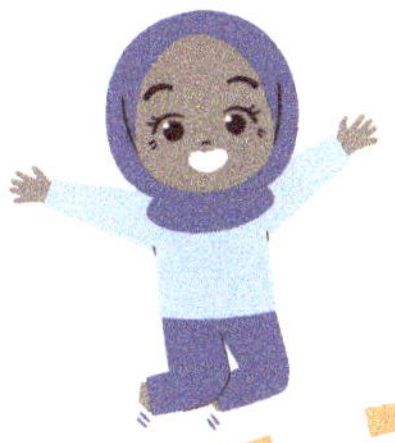

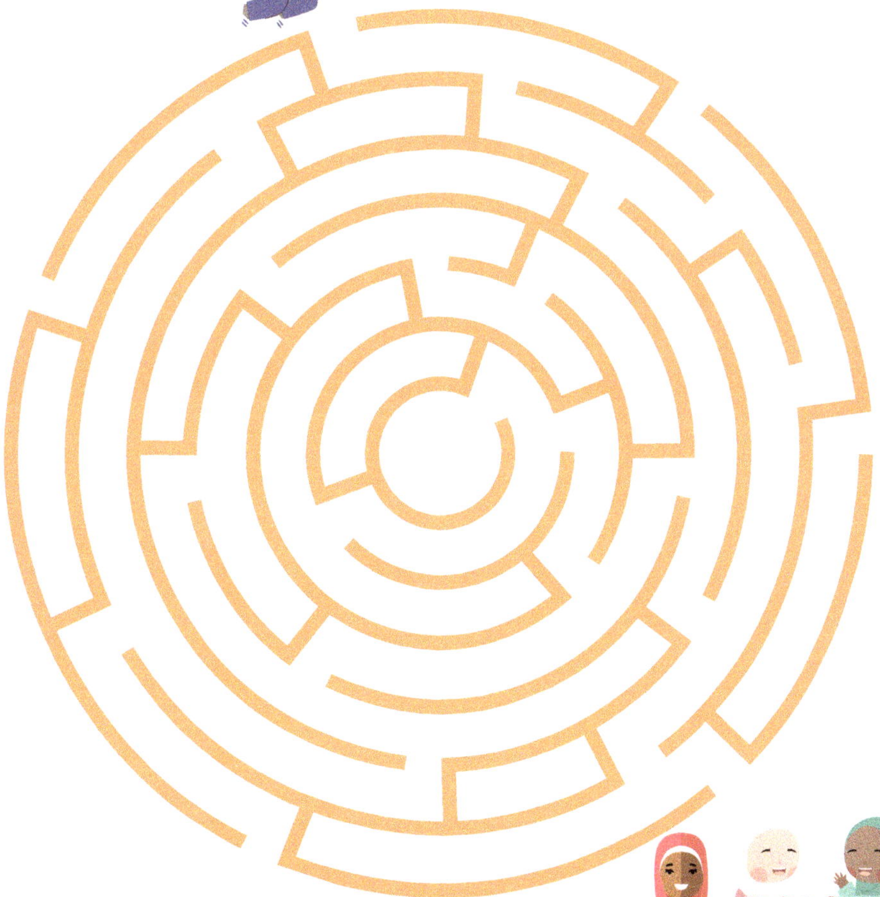

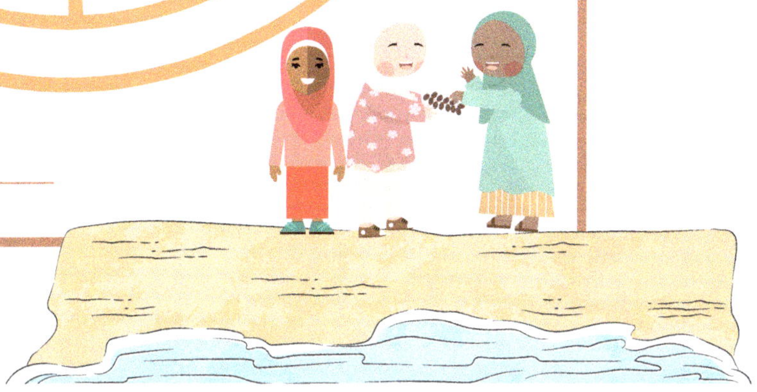

Name:_____

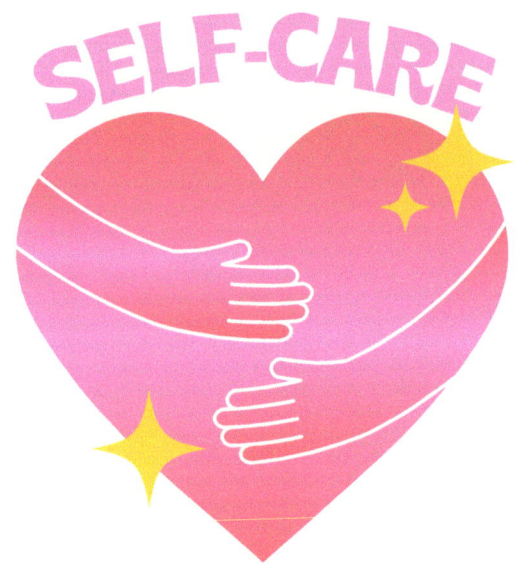

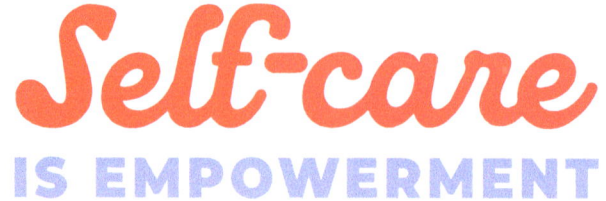

Wise Old Owl

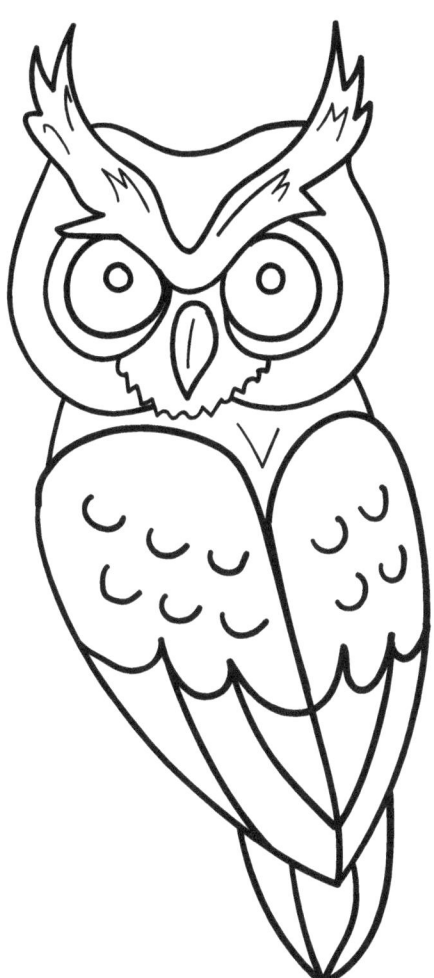

A wise old owl sat on an oak.
The more she saw the less she spoke.
The less she spoke the more she heard.
Why can't we all be like that wise old bird?

A theme is a message about life or human nature. What is the message or theme of this four-line poem?

In what ways do you think the poem makes a good point about the importance of having the wisdom to see and observe something without speaking?

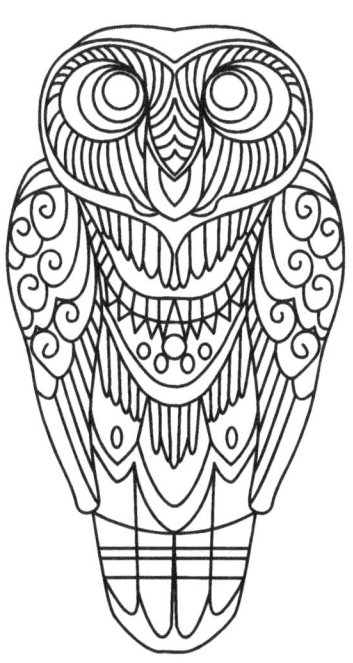

Date: _____

MINDFUL SENSES WALK

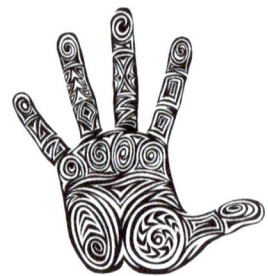

INSTRUCTION

Focus on what you see, hear, smell, touch, and possibly taste in your environment.
Read the questions. Write your answers in the boxes below.

I SEE..

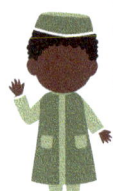

Look around and notice the colors, shapes, and patterns in your surroundings. Write down at least three things you see, and briefly describe what catches your eye.

I HEAR..

Listen carefully to the sounds around you. What can you hear?
Write down at least three distinct sounds, and note how they make you feel.

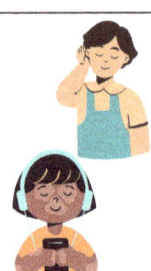

I SMELL..

Identify any scents in the air. What can you smell?
Describe at least three different smells and their characteristics.

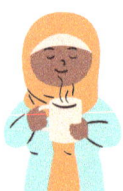

I FEEL..

Explore the sense of touch by reaching out and feeling various objects or surfaces. Describe the textures and sensations you experience when touching things like leaves, rocks, or tree bark.

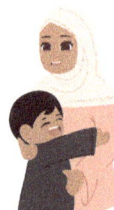

OVERCOME ANGER

3 Steps to Calm Down

1) Walk away from the person or object.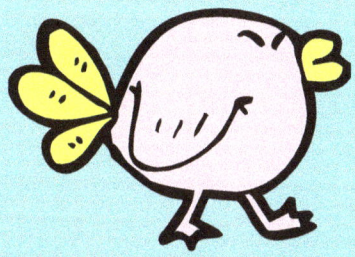

2) Concentrate on your breathing and count from 10 to 1.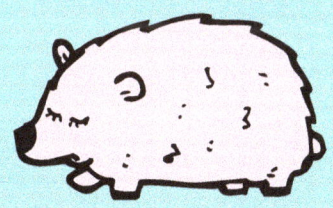

3) Imagine yourself in a happy place.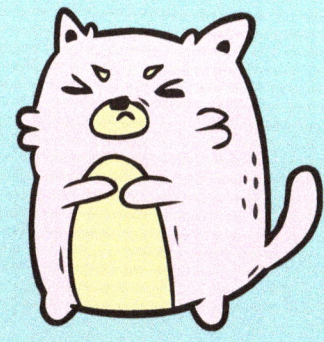

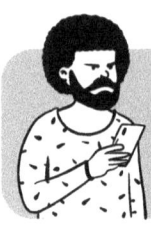
Feeling Angry
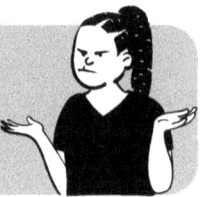

Anger looks different for everyone.

- What does your face look like when you're angry? Draw it

- Write and draw 4 things that make you feel angry.

　_____

　_____

　_____

　_____

- Write and draw 4 ways in which you express that you are angry.

　_____

　_____

　_____

　_____

COPING WITH ANGER

Write down five things that make you feel angry.

Write down five healthy coping skills.

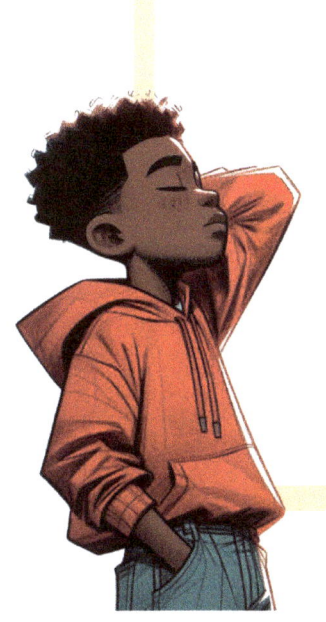

"The strong person is not the one who can wrestle well, but the strong person is the one who controls himself when angry."

(Sahih al-Bukhari, Hadith 6114)

Questions to Ask Yourself When Angry: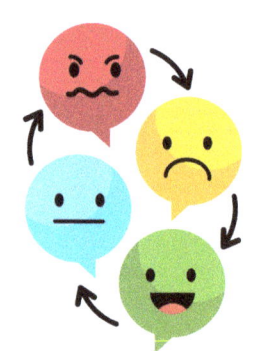

1. Why am I feeling angry?
   - Understanding the root cause can help calm the emotion.
2. Is this situation worth getting upset about?
   - Will it matter in the long run, or is it something small?
3. What will happen if I act on my anger?
   - Thinking about the consequences can prevent actions we might regret later.
4. How can I respond in a way that is fair and kind?
   - Focus on solutions instead of letting anger take over.
5. Would I want to be treated the way I'm about to act?
   - Remind yourself to treat others with respect, even when upset.

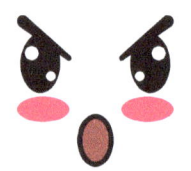 **Write message to yourself about managing anger.**

POWER IN YOUR BODY:
a secret trick to help your anger go away

Only do this activity when you find yourself angry.

Make a note of the time you felt anger. What happened?

"If one of you becomes angry while standing, he should sit down. If the anger goes away, fine. If not, he should lie down."

(Sunan Abi Dawood 4782)

Did you try sitting? How did you feel after sitting?

What it means, in a simple way:
1. When you get really angry, it's like your body fills up with lots of strong energy, and sometimes you might want to yell or do something not-so-nice.
2. Sitting down helps calm you because it makes your body feel more relaxed. It's hard to stay really angry when you're sitting!
3. If you still feel angry, lying down can help even more. It helps slow down your heart and makes you feel calmer and more peaceful.

Did you try lying down? How did you feel?

Lessons Learned:

CALM DOWN BY CHECKING YOUR PULSE AND USING SLOW, DEEP BREATHS TO LOWER YOUR HEART RATE

Step-by-Step Instructions:

1. **Find Your Pulse:**
   - Use two fingers to lightly press on your wrist or the side of your neck to feel your heartbeat.

2. **Check Your Heart Rate:**
   - Count your heartbeats for 15 seconds, then multiply that number by 4 to get your heart rate in beats per minute (BPM)

 3. Use This Heart Rate Chart to Guide Your Breathing:

Heart Rate (BPM)	How You Might Feel	Breathing Tips
60-80 BPM	Calm, normal breathing	Keep breathing slowly and deeply.
80-100 BPM	Slightly stressed or anxious	Inhale deeply for 4 seconds, exhale for 6.
100-120 BPM	Angry or upset	Breathe in for 4 seconds, hold for 4, then exhale for 6. Repeat.
120+ BPM	Very angry or panicked	Stop, sit or lie down, breathe deeply and slowly, focusing on calming your heart.

4. **Focus on Your Breathing:**
   - Try deep belly breathing (inhaling slowly through your nose, holding briefly, then exhaling through your mouth) to bring your heart rate back down.

5. **Recheck Your Pulse:**
   - After a few minutes of deep breathing, check your pulse again. Notice if your heart rate has slowed, and continue deep breathing until you feel calmer.

Name: _____   Date: _____

Emotions

Look at the pictures and circle the correct words

☀️	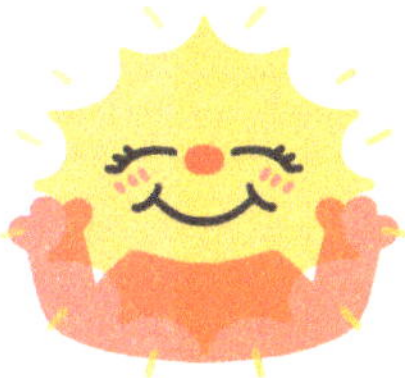 NERVOUS / HAPPY	🤢	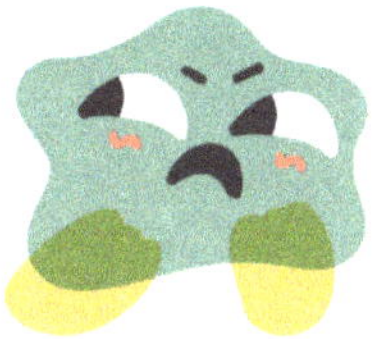 DISGUSTED / CALM
😢	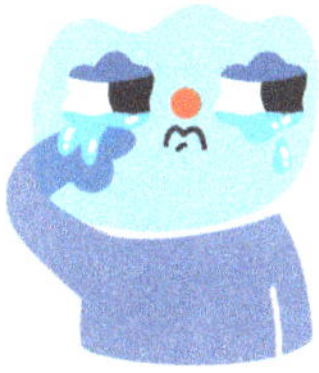 SAD / ANGRY	☀️	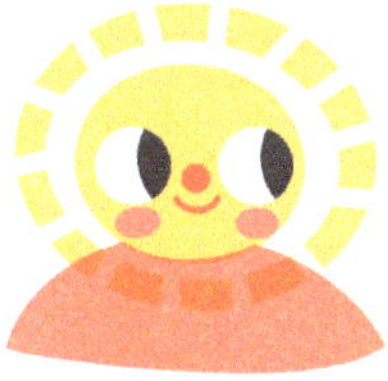 HAPPY / SURPRISED
❓	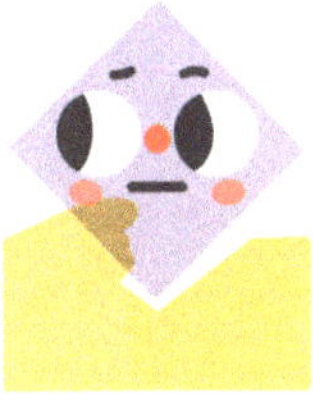 CONFUSED / JOYFUL	😰	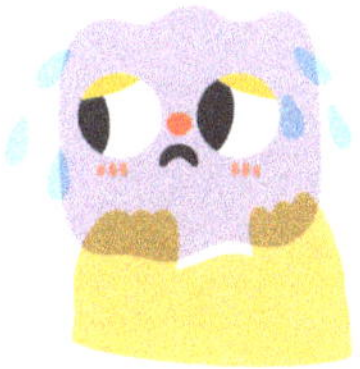 GRATEFUL / NERVOUS
🔥	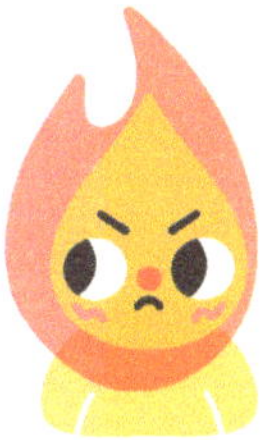 NERVOUS / ANGRY	😔	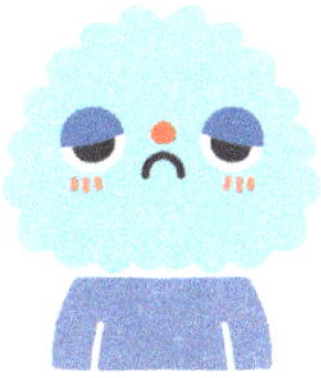 FURIOUS / LONELY
🌼	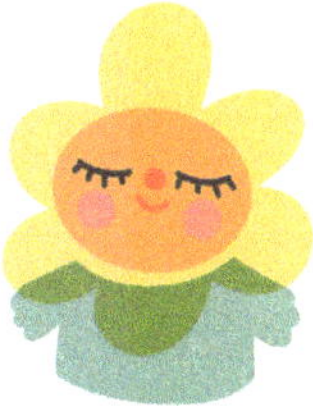 CALM / DISGUSTED	😴	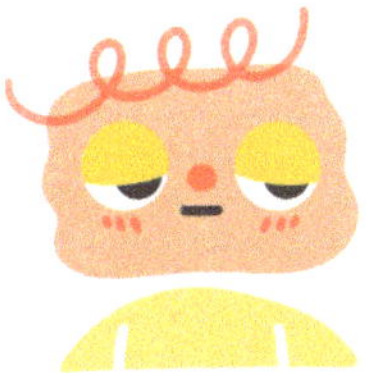 SLEEPY / NERVOUS

TEMPER TEMPER

THINGS TO DO WHEN I'M ANGRY

1. Go to a quiet place.

2. Take deep breaths.

3. Count backwards slowly.

4. Talk about why I feel angry.

5. Doodle circles on my notebook.

6. Wait and cool off until I feel calm.

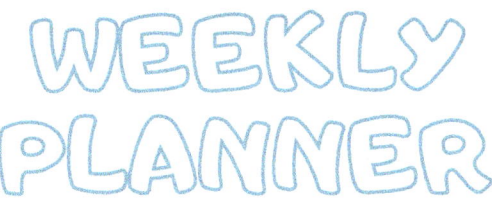

WEEKLY PLANNER

WHAT DO YOU WANT TO ACCOMPLISH THIS WEEK? WORK ON YOUR PASSIONS DAILY. WHAT WILL YOU DO EACH DAY? WRITE IT DOWN HERE.

MONDAY

TUESDAY

WEDNESDAY

THURSDAY

FRIDAY

SATURDAY

NOTES AND IDEA

....

....

....

....

إِنَّ ٱلْحَسَنَٰتِ يُذْهِبْنَ ٱلسَّيِّئَاتِ

"Surely, good deeds erase bad deeds."

Write or draw a picture to share ways you can be kind to erase bad deeds.

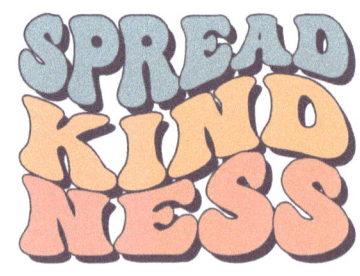

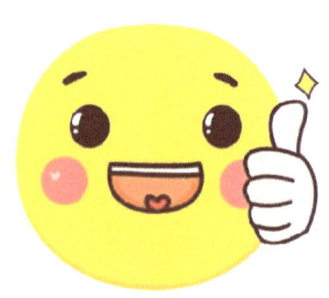

Daily check in

DATE _____

TODAY I'M GRATEFUL FOR
- _____
- _____
- _____

TODAY'S AFFIRMATION
_____

TODAY I FELT
_____

WHAT I WANT TO REMEMBER ABOUT TODAY
_____

WHAT WAS THE BEST THING ABOUT TODAY?
_____

THINGS I DID TODAY
- _____
- _____
- _____
- _____

PEOPLE I MET TODAY
_____

MY RANKING OF TODAY

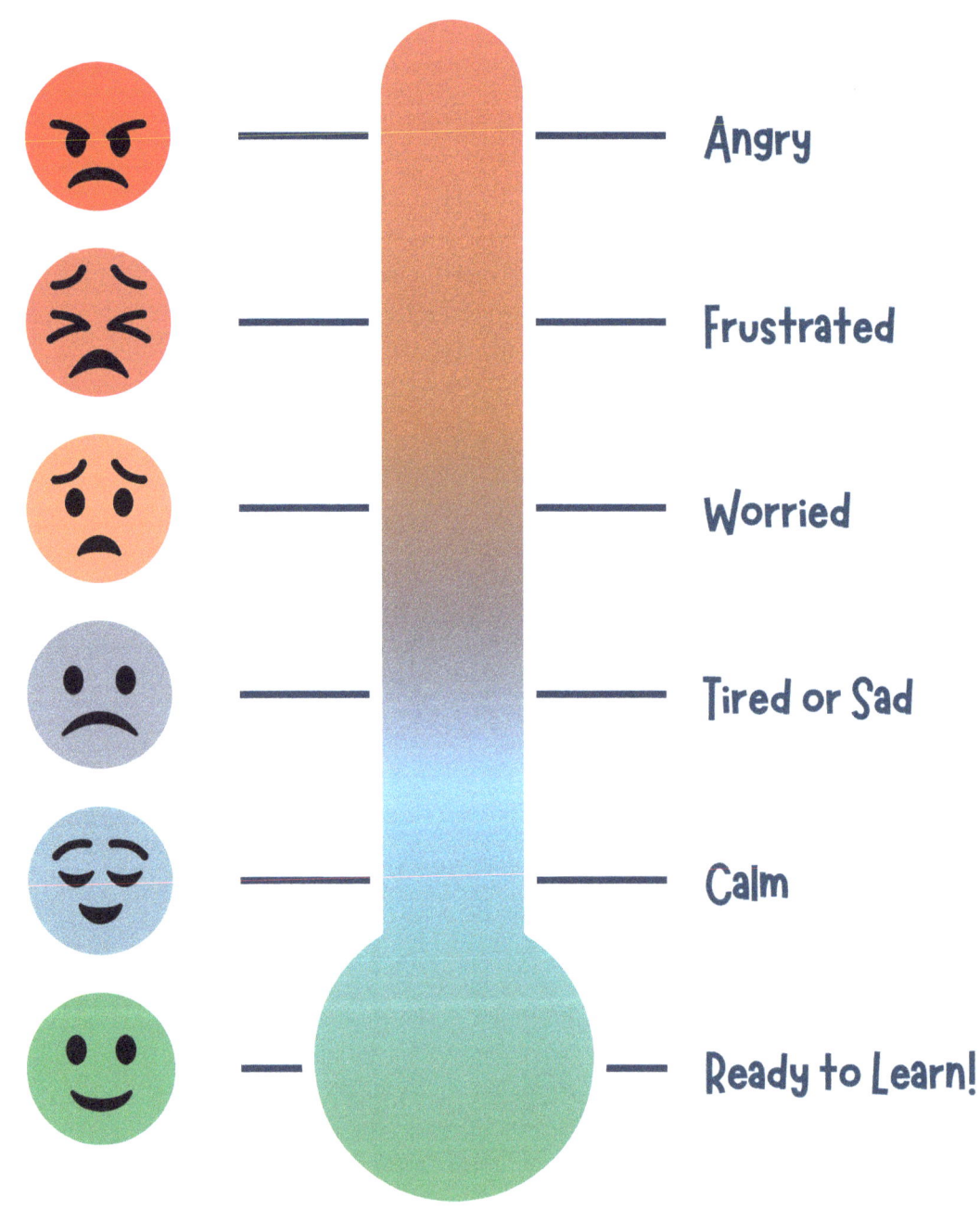

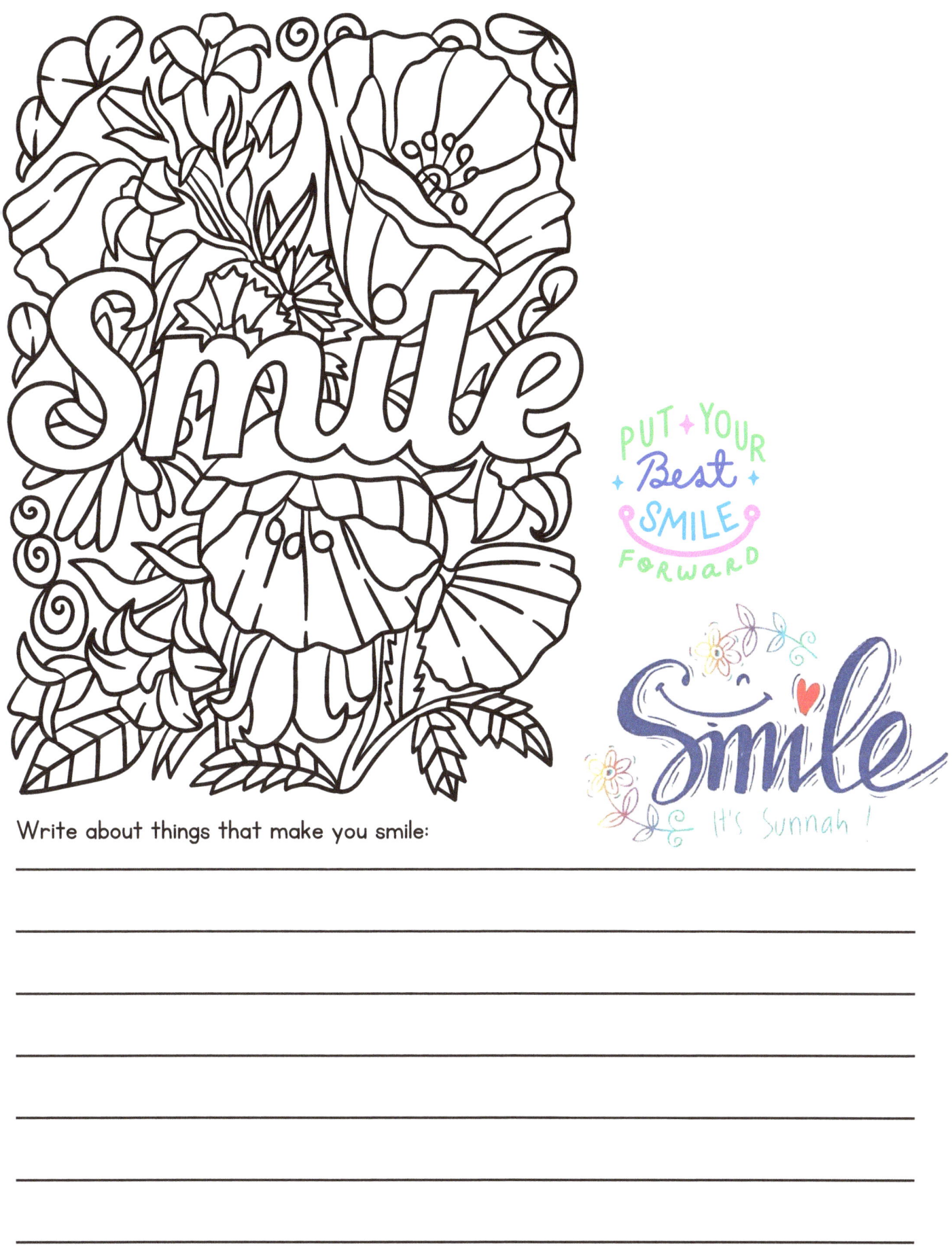

Write about things that make you smile:
_____
_____
_____
_____
_____
_____
_____

THOUGHT CLOUDS

In the clouds, write words to describe your thoughts and feelings.

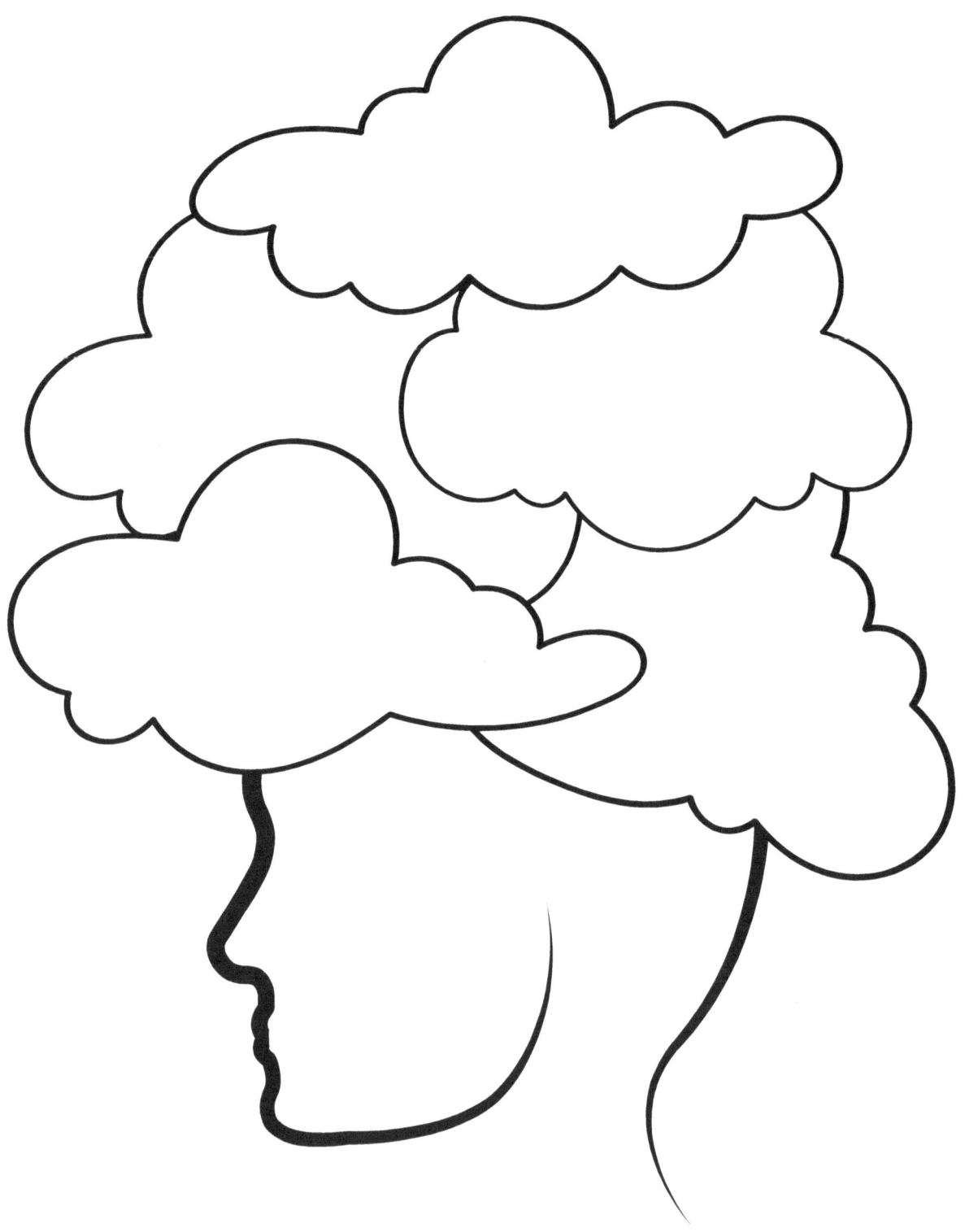

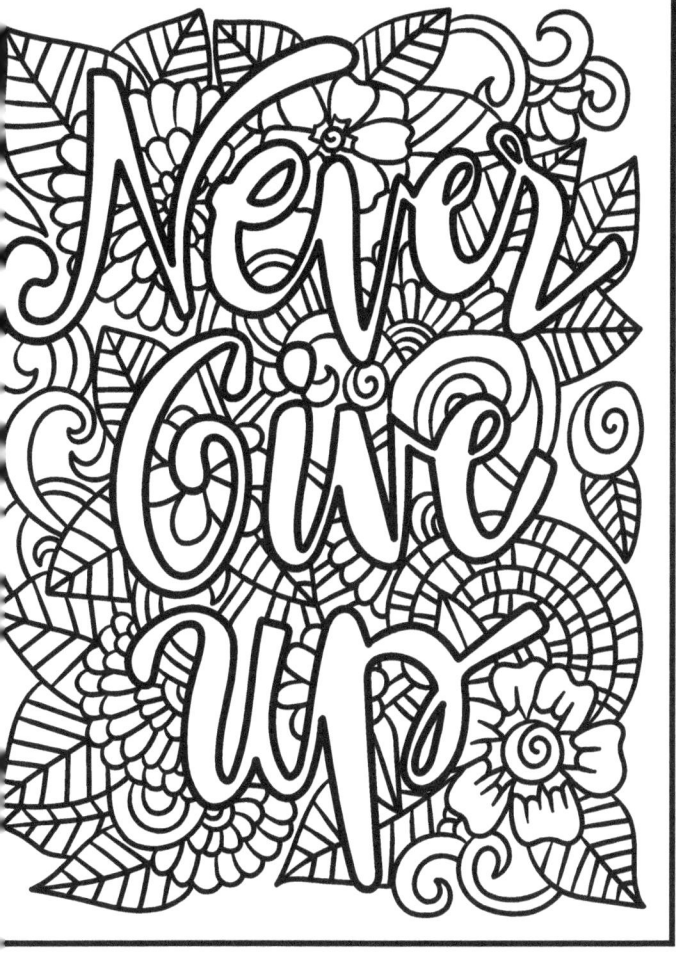

"Oh you who believe! Seek help with patient perseverance and prayer, for God is with those who patiently persevere."
(Qur'an 2:153)

Write about a time you demonstrated perseverance:

_____
_____
_____
_____
_____
_____
_____
_____
_____

Use a dictionary to define patient and perseverance. What is the difference between the two words?

_____
_____
_____
_____
_____
_____

Name: _____   Date: _____

Today's REFLECTION

Today is:

How I feel about today:

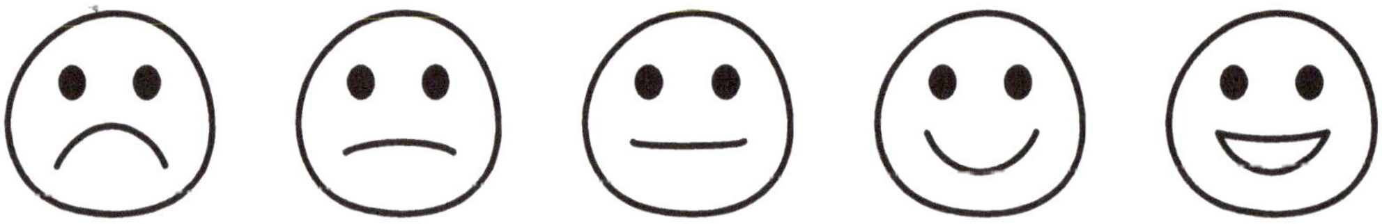

😞 😐 🙂 😊 😃

My act of kindness:

Reason for my rating

_____
_____
_____
_____
_____

Something new I learned today:

_____
_____
_____

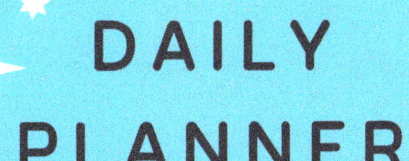

DAILY PLANNER

Date
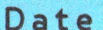

MON TUE WED THU FRI SAT SUN

BREAKFAST

LUNCH

DINNER

GOALS

REMEMBER!

TO DO LIST
....
....
....
....
....

NOTES

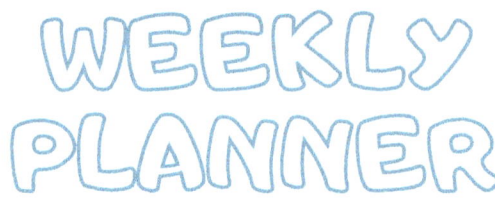

WEEKLY PLANNER

WHAT DO YOU WANT TO ACCOMPLISH THIS WEEK? WORK ON YOUR PASSIONS DAILY. WHAT WILL YOU DO EACH DAY? WRITE IT DOWN HERE.

MONDAY

TUESDAY

WEDNESDAY

THURSDAY

FRIDAY

SATURDAY

NOTES AND IDEA

Read your heart out!

Reading is like a superpower!

Reading helps you feel better when you're sad or worried because stories can take you to new places or teach you how others face challenges, which can be comforting.

Reading is super fun because you can explore magical lands, meet interesting characters, and learn amazing things you never knew!

Reading is revolutionary!

It can change the way you see the world and help you grow smarter and stronger. With every book, you're building a better, braver version of yourself, ready to make the world a better place

READ A CHAPTER OF A BOOK OR A SHORT STORY. Once you're done, here are some fun questions to think about and answer:

1. Who is the main character? What do they like to do or what makes them special?

2. Where does the story happen? Is it a real place or somewhere imaginary?

3. What problem does the character face? How do they try to solve it?

4. Did anything in the story surprise you? What part?

5. What was your favorite part of the story? Why did you like it?

6. If you could be one character from the story, who would you be? Why?

7. What do you think happens next? Imagine what could happen if the story continued!

Reading is like going on an adventure! Let's see where your story takes you.

Date: _____

Do you like...?

1) Look at the chart. Complete the second column with the names of the vegetables.

2) Now, complete the chart about you. Circle the vegetables you have never eaten or tased. Put a tick for the vegetables you like, or an X if you don't like it.

		Me	how I will include in my diet

Fruit Puzzle

Place the names of the fruits shown in the pictures into the puzzle using the clues.

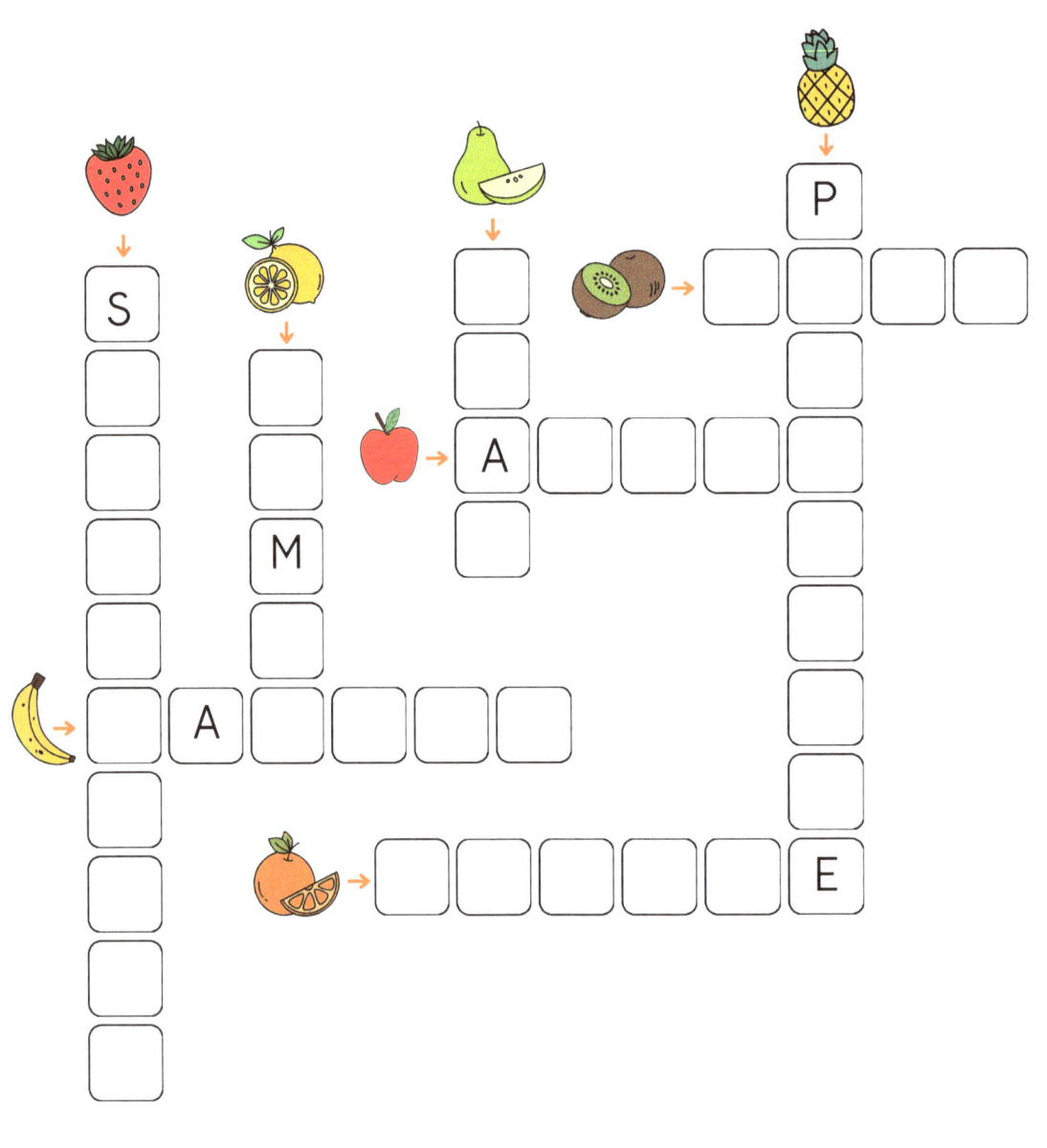

Self-Reflection PMI

STAR RATING

How successful was I in achieving my desired result?

FEELING

How do I feel about my results?

PLUS

What were my strengths? In which areas was I most successful?

MINUS

What were my weaknesses? In which areas was I least successful?

IMPROVE

What are some specific strategies or activities I can undertake to improve particular skills for next time?

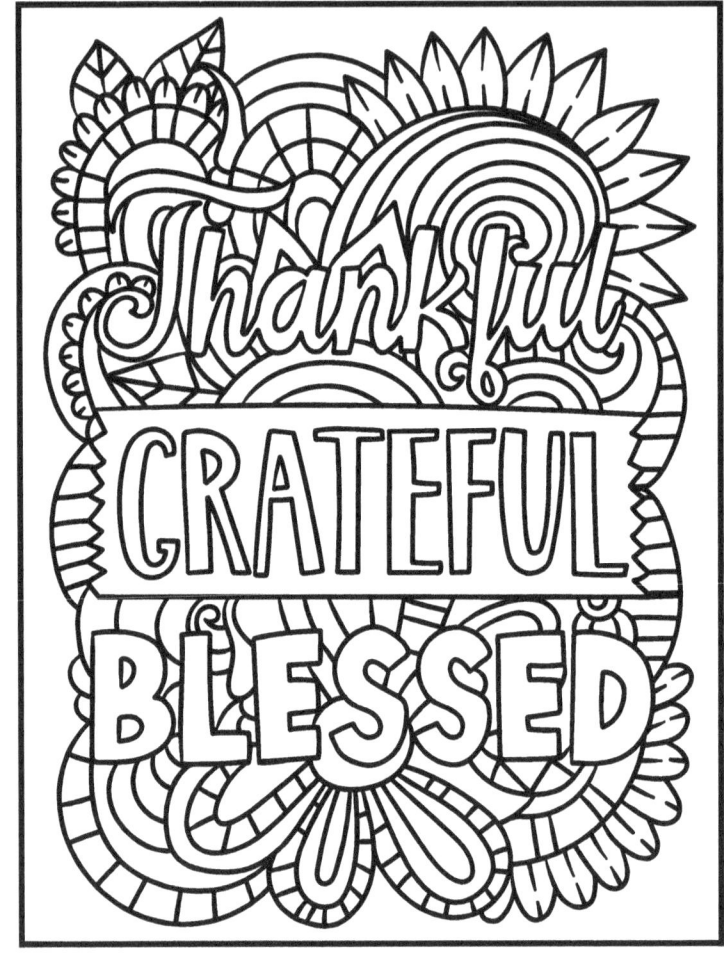

"If you are grateful,
I will certainly
give more..."
(Qur'an 14:7)

Write about ways you can show your gratitude.
_____
_____
_____
_____
_____
_____
_____
_____
_____
_____

Use a dictionary to define grateful. What makes you grateful?

_____
_____
_____
_____
_____
_____
_____
_____

I SPY COLORING PAGE

Name, write down and color ten things you can spy in the picture.

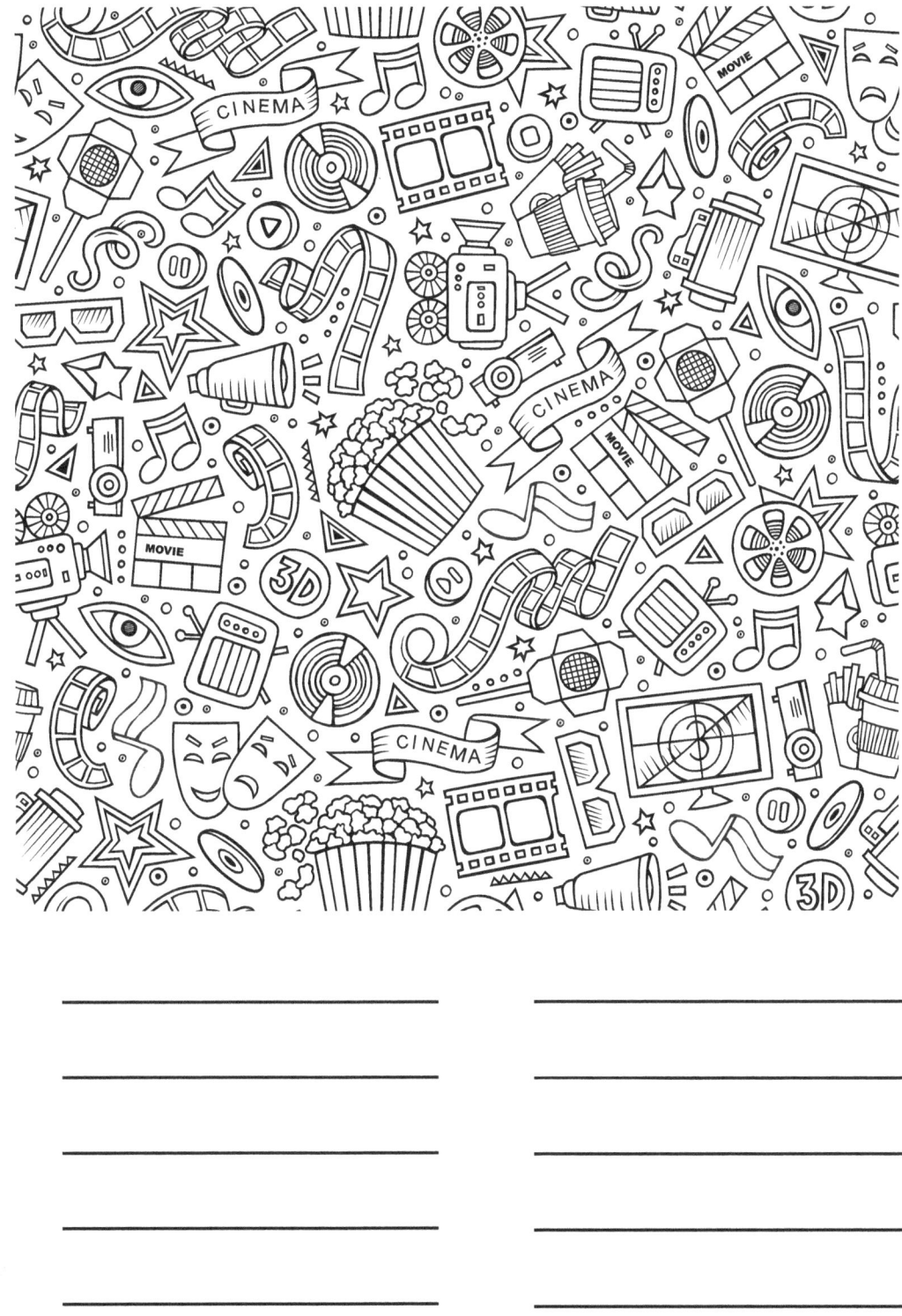

Write about any of the items. Writing can be fun~

_____   _____

_____   _____

_____   _____

_____   _____

_____   _____

Check-in

Feelings can be overwhelming for us and that is completely okay! Check-in with your own feelings and see if you can figure them out. Then, fill this container with feeling colors to show how much of each you have right now.

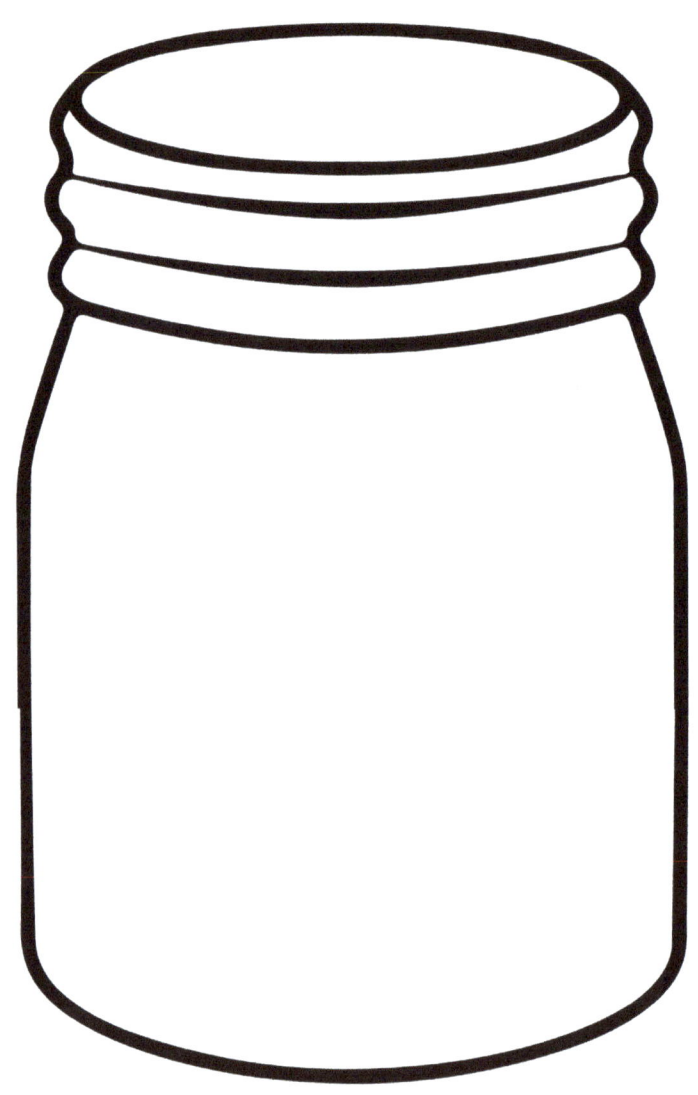

Angry	Happy	Sad
Nervous	Excited	Calm

Sculpture Research

Research the history behind the sculpture.

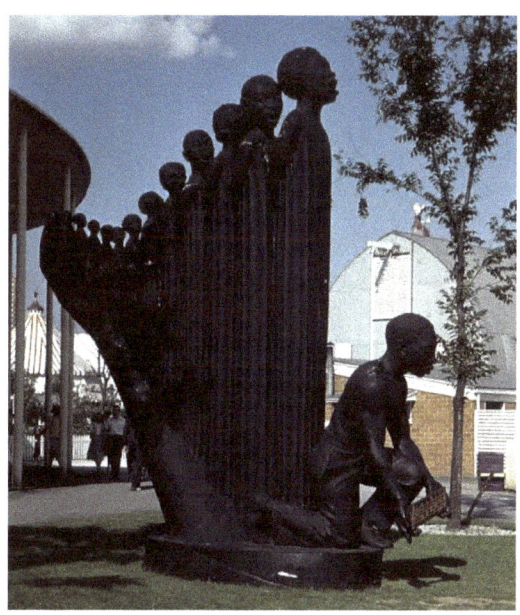

Analysis

Share your personal thoughts and feelings about the chosen sculpture.

Write your answer here...

Origin

Title: "The Harp"

Year Made:

Materials:

Artist: Augusta Savage

History

Explain any historical events or influences that might have impacted the creation of this sculpture.

Write your answer here...

MINDFULNESS

Some activities I can do to help me relax include:

Some music I can listen to includes:

Some things I can focus on and think about are:

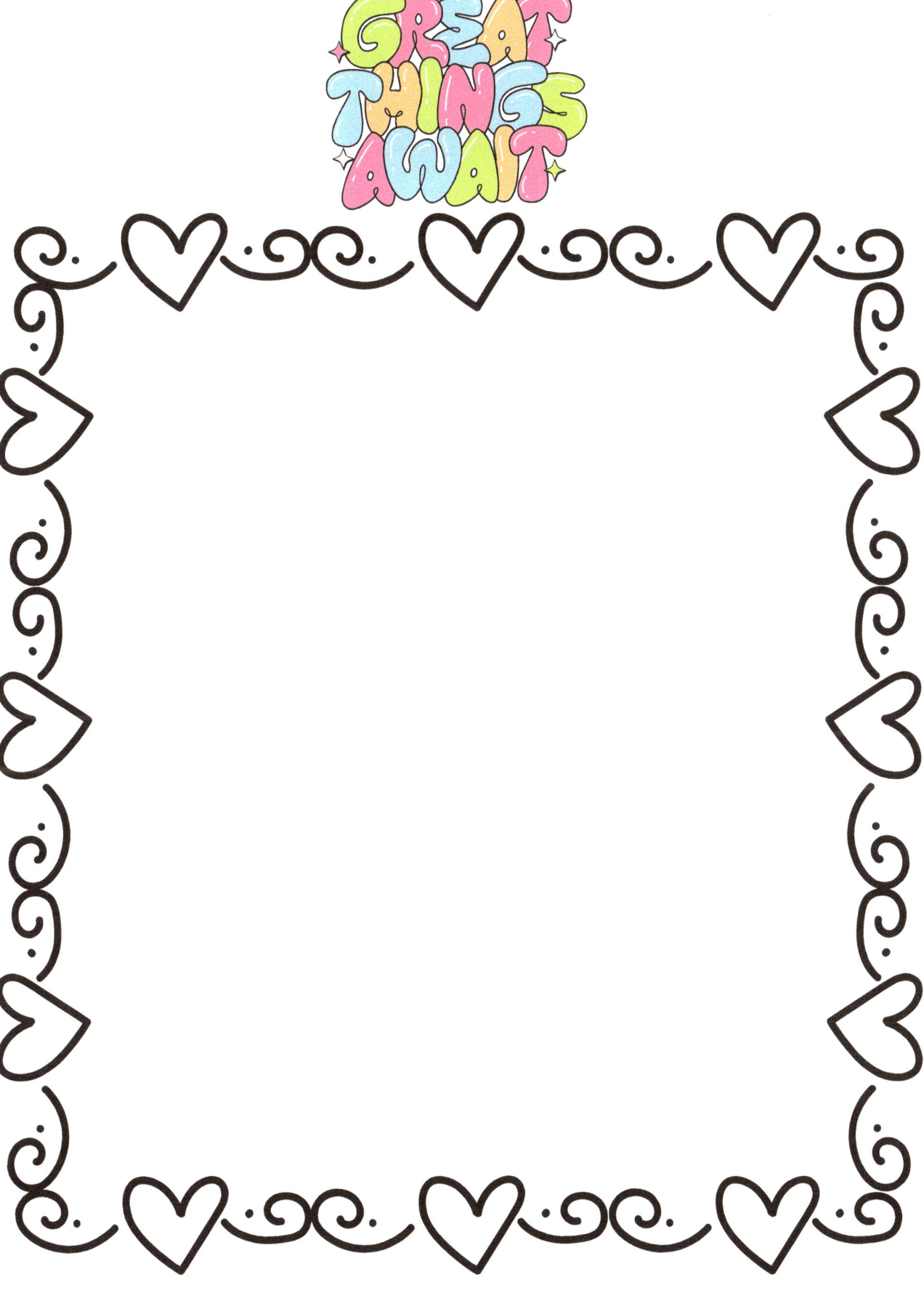

See and Write

Which objects are in the jar? Write the objects' names in the list.

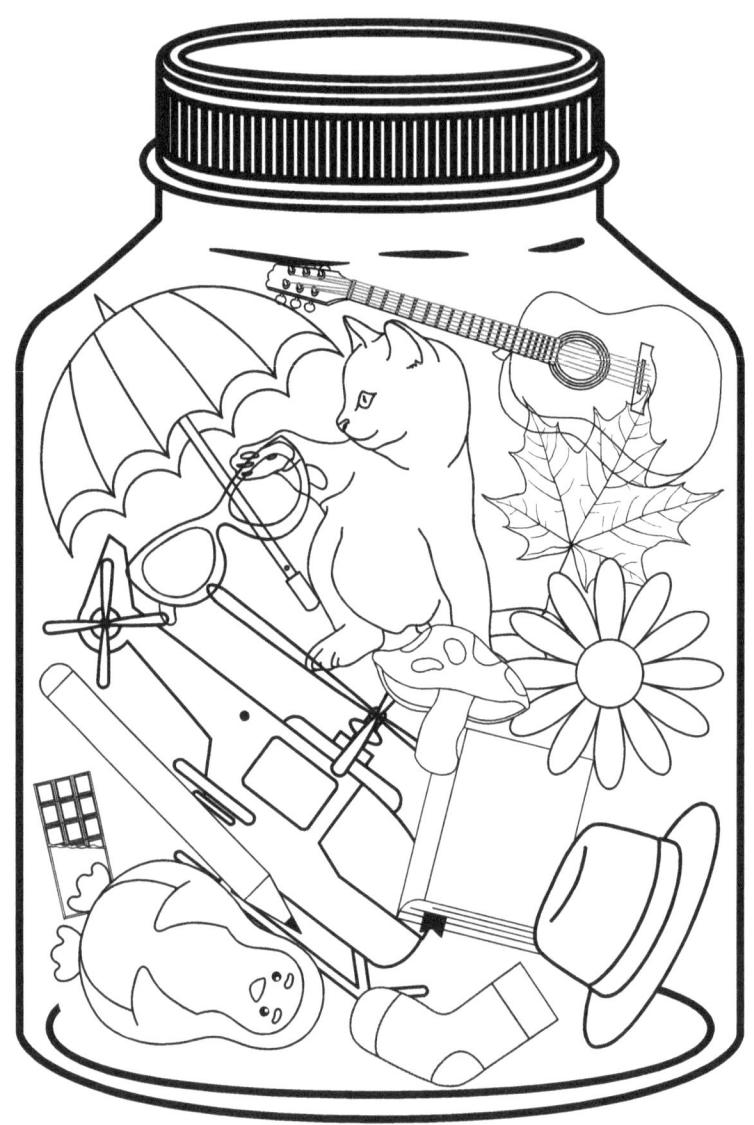

1. ....
2. ....
3. ....
4. ....
5. ....
6. ....
7. ....
8. ....
9. ....
10. ....
11. ....
12. ....
13. ....
14. ....

Art Comparison

Use the spaces below to compare the two different works of art.

Artwork 1

Title:

Artist:

Year Made:

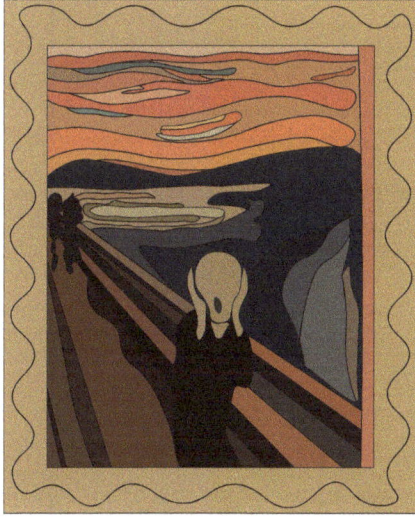

Similarities

- What makes these two pieces of art similar?

Write your answer here.....

Differences

- What makes these two pieces of art different?

Write your answer here.....

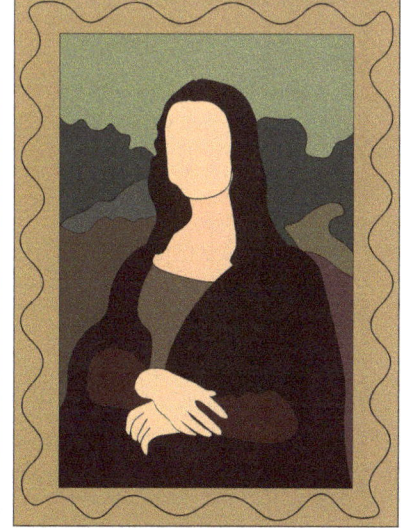

Artwork 2

Title:

Artist:

Year Made:

Ramadan Activity

Help Samir find his way to the iftar meal.

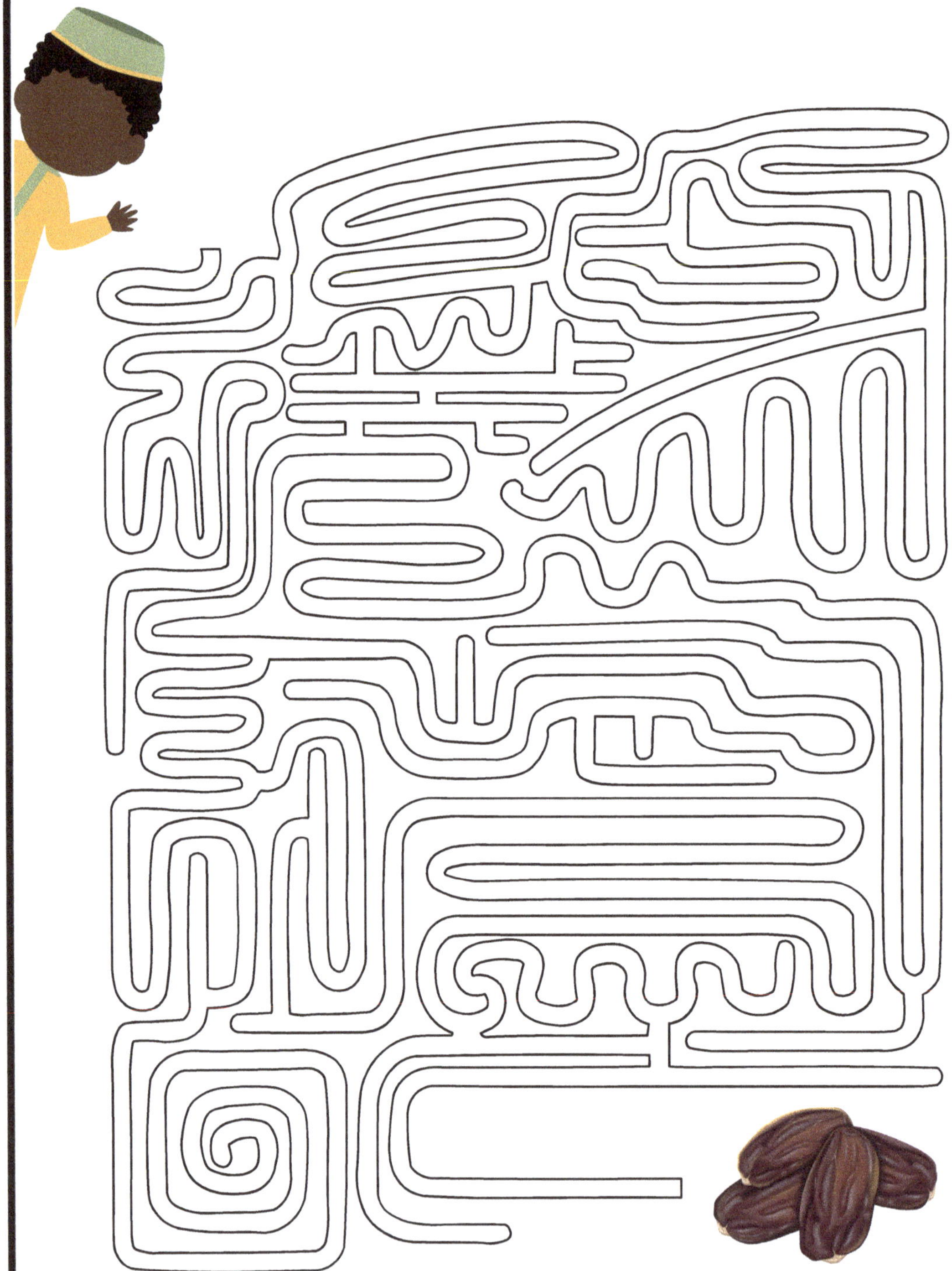

HABIT TRACKER

	M	T	W	T	F	S	S
WATER	○	○	○	○	○	○	○
JOYFUL MOVEMENT	○	○	○	○	○	○	○
READ	○	○	○	○	○	○	○
WRITING	○	○	○	○	○	○	○
HEALTHY EATING	○	○	○	○	○	○	○
SLEEP	○	○	○	○	○	○	○

TO DO LIST

- ....
- ....
- ....
- ....
- ....
- ....
- ....
- ....
- ....
- ....

NOTES

- ....
- ....
- ....
- ....
- ....
- ....
- ....
- ....
- ....
- ....

Name: _____ Date: _____

Today's REFLECTION

Today is: _____

How I feel about today:

☹ 😐 🙂 😀 😃

Reason for my rating

My act of kindness:

_____
_____
_____
_____
_____
_____

Something new I learned today:

_____
_____
_____

How to choose the best friends:

When I see them, they remind me about The Almighty.
When I sit with them, my faith (Iman) increases.
When I speak to them, my knowledge about spirituality
and religious convictions increases.
They are the ones pushing me towards Paradise and Goodness.
They are my companions in this world and the hereafter.
They are worth more than anything and everything
this world can possibly offer.

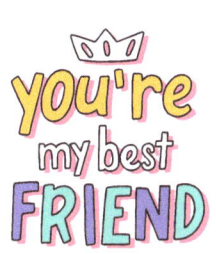

Who are your real friends?
How do you count on one another?

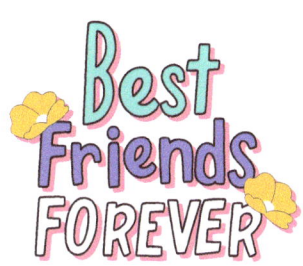

Vision Board

(Day):   (Month):   (Year):

(Remember)
CULTIVATING GRATITUDE IS A POWERFUL PRACTICE THAT CAN POSITIVELY IMPACT YOUR MINDSET AND OVERALL WELL-BEING. ENJOY THIS RITUAL, AND WATCH HOW IT CONTRIBUTES TO FULFILLED LIFE.

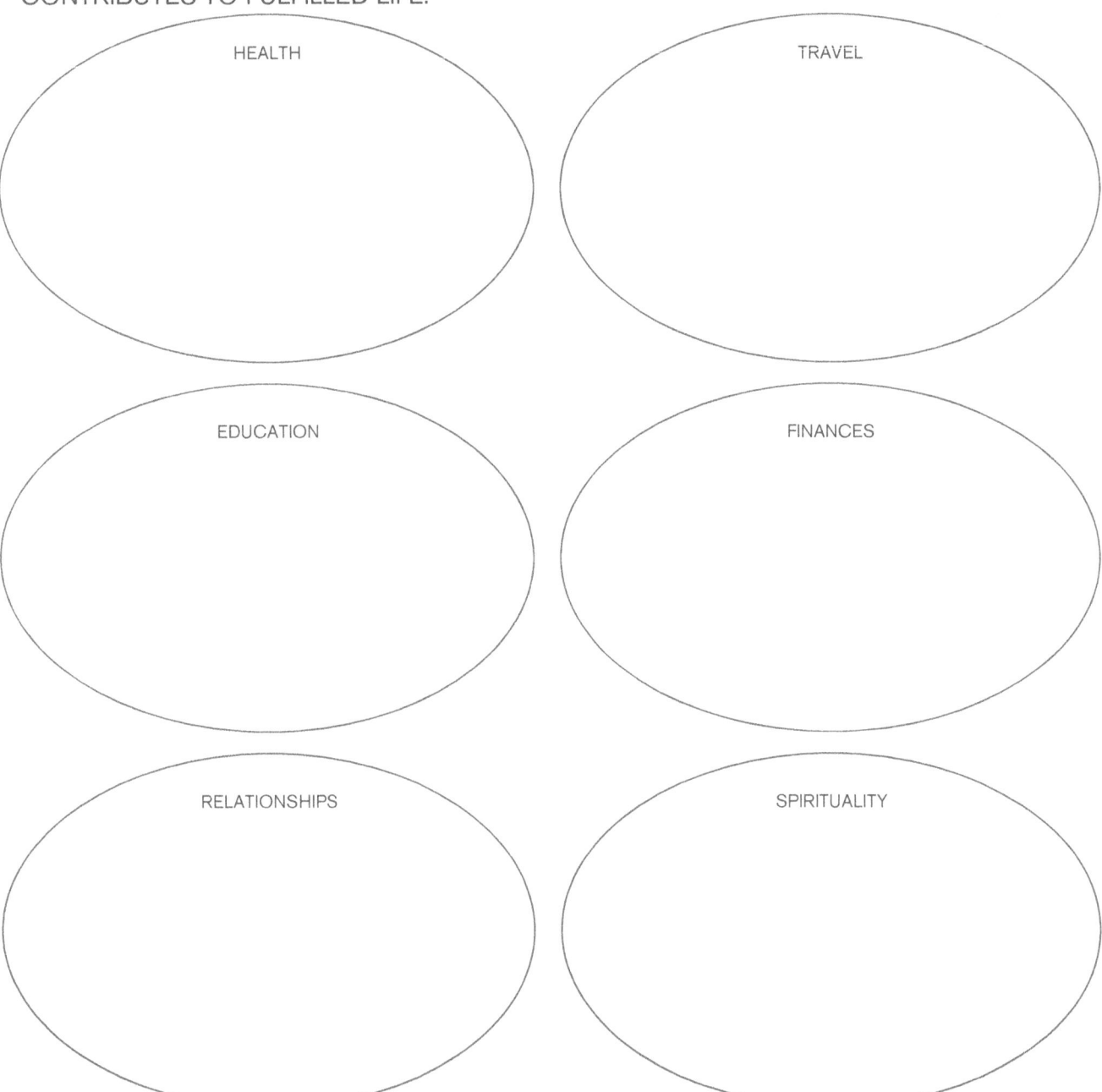

INDEED, WE CREATED HUMANS IN THE BEST FORM
(Qur'an 95:4)

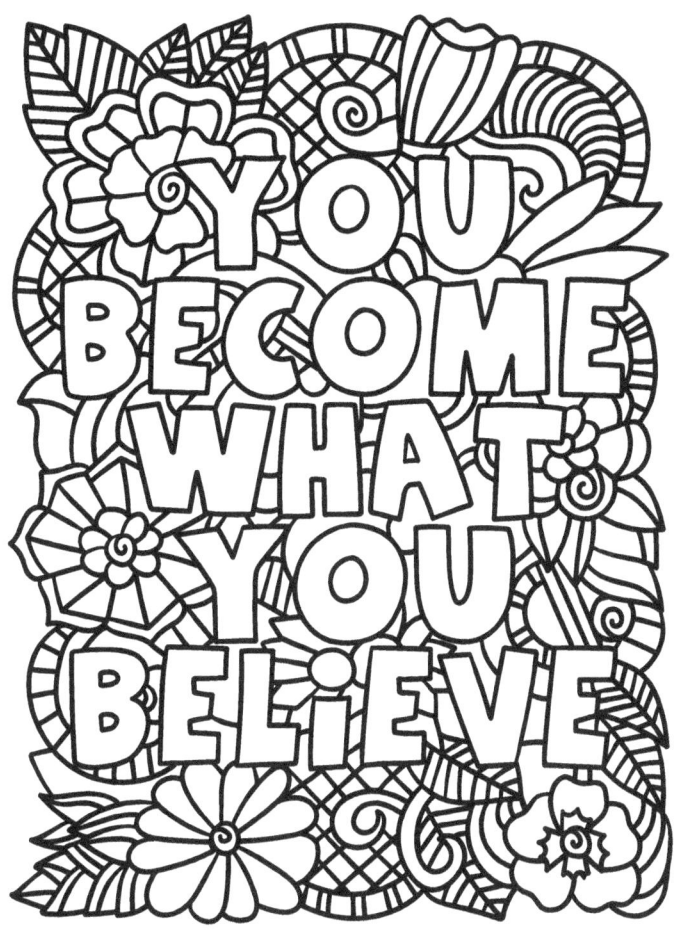

What do you believe your best form is?

Write down your personal goals for the future:

_____

_____

_____

_____

_____

_____

_____

_____

My Own Comic

Draw your comic and add text to accompany your illustrations.

1. Choose Your Characters
Who will your comic be about? It can be a superhero, an animal, or even you! Give them a name and think about what they like to do.

2. Think of a Problem or Adventure
Every comic needs a fun story! What challenge does your character face? Maybe they need to save the day, find a treasure, or help a friend.

4. Add Speech Bubbles and Words
Inside the panels, draw your characters and give them speech bubbles for what they're saying. You can also add sound effects like "BAM!" or "ZAP!" for action!

3. Draw Your Panels
A comic has boxes called panels that show different parts of the story. Start by drawing a few panels (like little windows) on your paper. Each panel shows a new part of the story.

Drawing and making comic art can be healing
It helps you express your feelings in a fun way. When you draw, you can turn your worries, sadness, or even happiness into pictures.

5. End with a Fun Conclusion
How does the adventure end? Did your character solve the problem or learn something new?

Creating characters and stories lets you share your emotions without having to say a lot of words. It's like talking to your heart through art! Plus, making comics can make you feel proud and calm, like you're putting your thoughts and feelings in a safe place.

Art is a way to feel better and have fun at the same time!

My Own Comic

Draw your comic and add text to accompany your illustrations.

Being your best self..........................

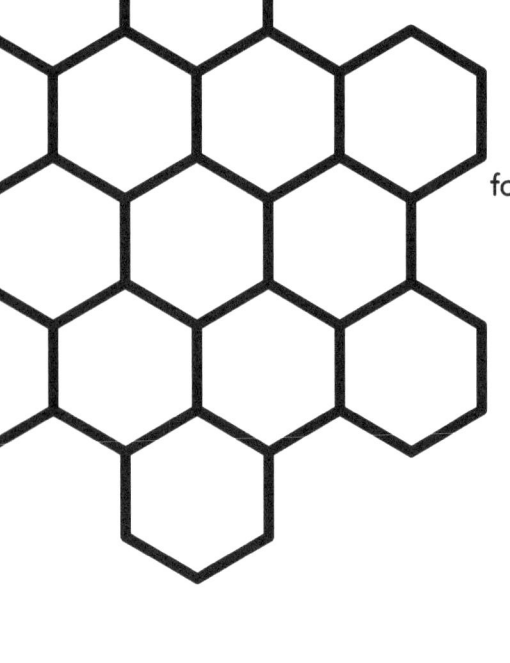

"It is not righteousness that you turn your faces towards East or West.
But it is righteousness to believe in Allah and the Last Day,
And the Angels, and the Book, and the Messengers;
To spend of your substance, out of love for Him,
For your kin, for orphans, for the needy,
for the wayfarer, for those who ask, and for the ransom of slaves;
To be steadfast in prayer
And give in charity;
To fulfill the contracts which you have made;
And to be firm and patient, in pain and adversity
And throughout all periods of panic.
Such are the people of truth, the God-fearing.

Qur'an 2:177

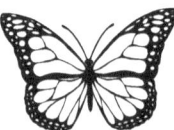

DAILY PLANNER

Date
....

MON TUE WED THU FRI SAT SUN

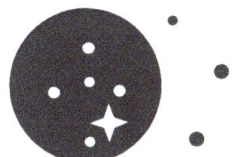
BREAKFAST

LUNCH

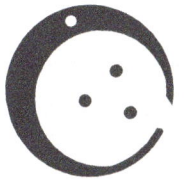
DINNER

GOALS

REMEMBER!

TO DO LIST

....
....
....
....
....

NOTES

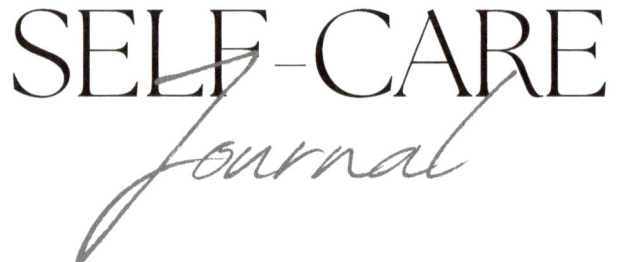

DATE: / /

S M T W T F S

TODAY I'M GRATEFUL FOR:

1.
2.
3.

WATER INTAKE

1 2 3 4 5 6 7 8 (Glass)

MOOD

ANGRY TIRED SAD HAPPY EXCITED

TODAY'S AFFIRMATION

NOTES/REMINDER:

FOR TOMORROW

resilience

Verily, with every difficulty there is relief.
Verily, with every difficulty there is relief.

Qur'an 94:5–6

- Write the word resilience 25 times.
- Each time you write the word tell yourself how brilliant you are and how you are able to get through difficult times.

Optimism
Self-belief
Control of Self
Willingness to Adapt
Willingness to Be Flexible → *Resilience*
Ability to Solve Problems
Emotional Awareness
Social Support
Sense of Humor

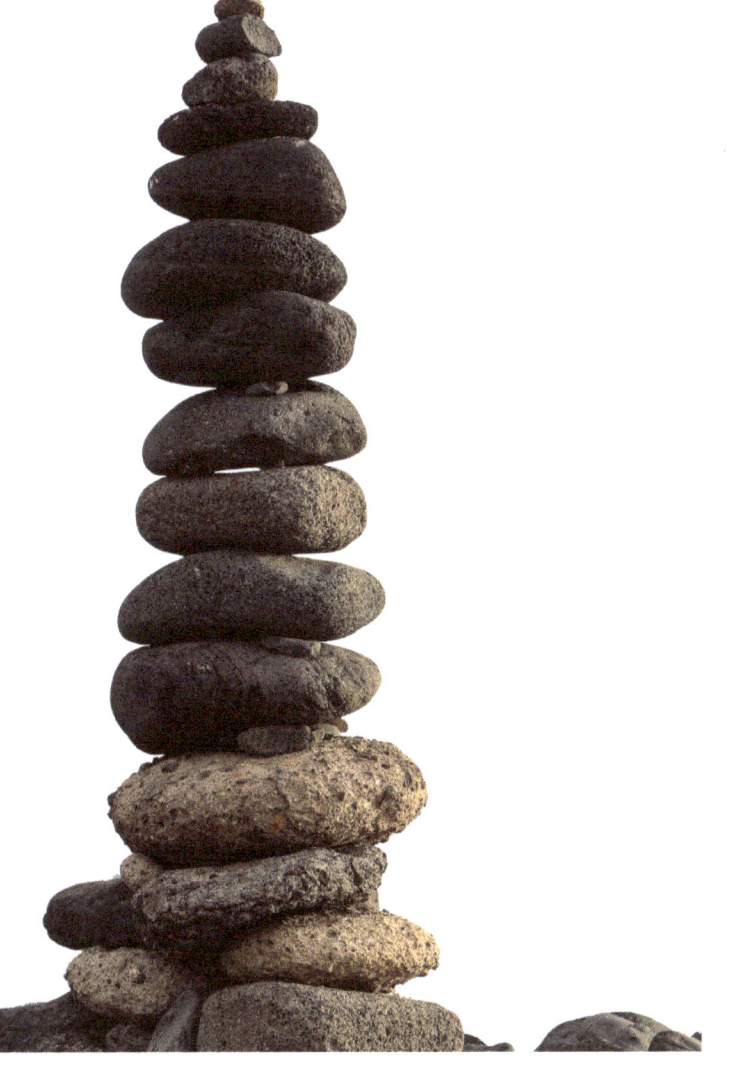

Name: _____   Date: _____

Today's REFLECTION

Today is:

How I feel about today:

😞 😐 🙂 😊 😃

My act of kindness:

Reason for my rating

_____
_____
_____
_____
_____
_____

Something new I learned today:

_____
_____
_____

MINDFUL SCAVENGER HUNT

We can practice mindfulness outdoors by observing what we see, hear, smell, taste, and feel. See how many of the following you can do or find.

1 Notice the weather. Is it sunny or cloudy? How does the air feel (warm, cold, windy)?

2 Find a tree and touch the bark and leaves. What do they feel like?

3 Smell a flower or a plant. How would you describe the scent?

4 Observe a bug without disturbing it.

5 Notice what you hear outside. Do you hear the wind, birds, or insects?

6 Look for seeds, pods, or nuts. How many types can you find?

7 Lay on the ground. How does the earth feel beneath you? What do you see in the sky?

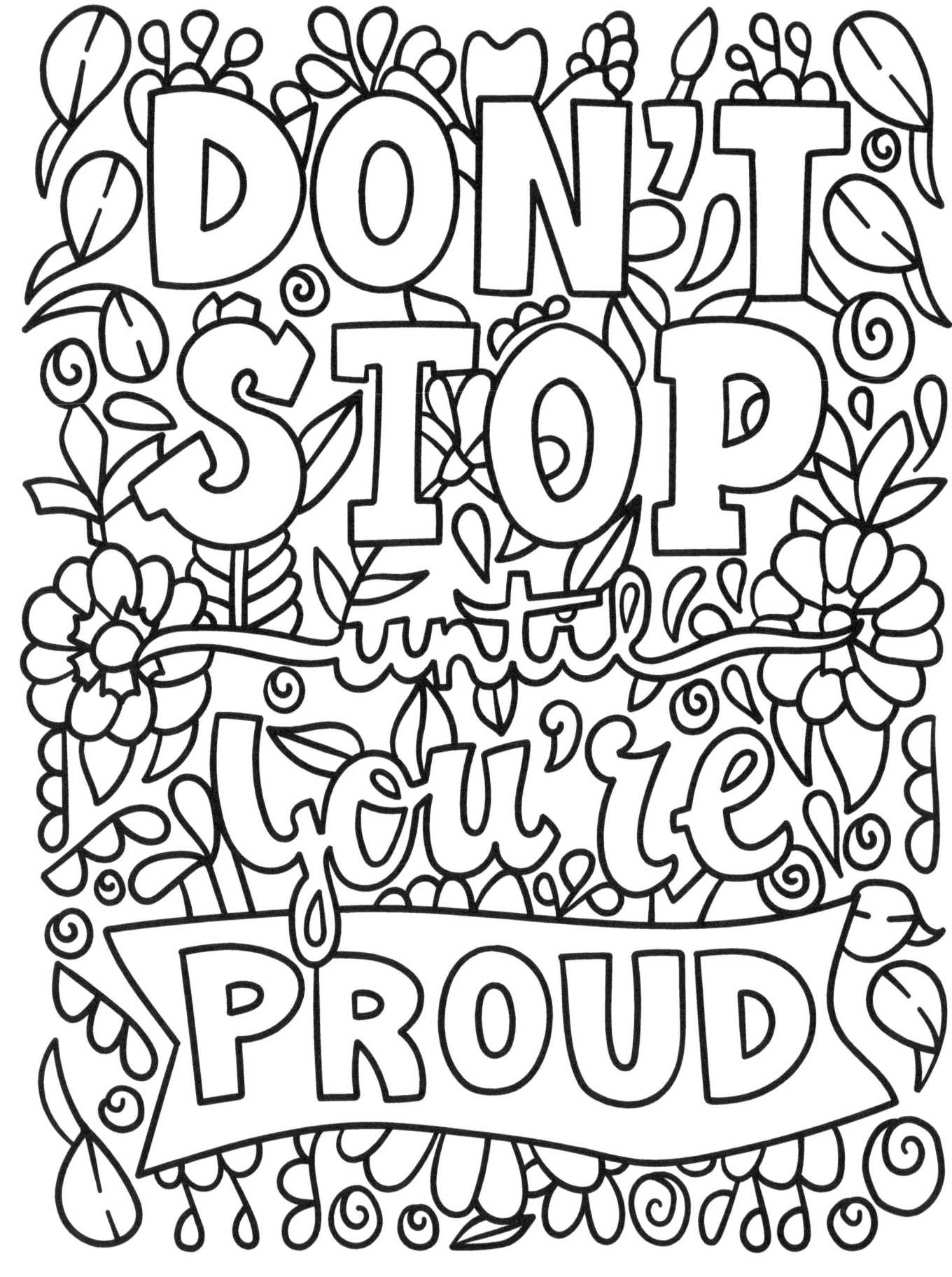

Daily Gratitude

3 things I'm grateful for today...

_____
_____
_____
_____
_____
_____

What can I learn from today's experiences?

_____
_____
_____
_____
_____
_____

Date:

Date: _____

What does "healing" mean to you?

_____
_____
_____
_____
_____
_____
_____
_____
_____
_____
_____
_____
_____
_____
_____
_____
_____
_____
_____

See and Write

Which objects are in the jar? Write the objects' names in the list.

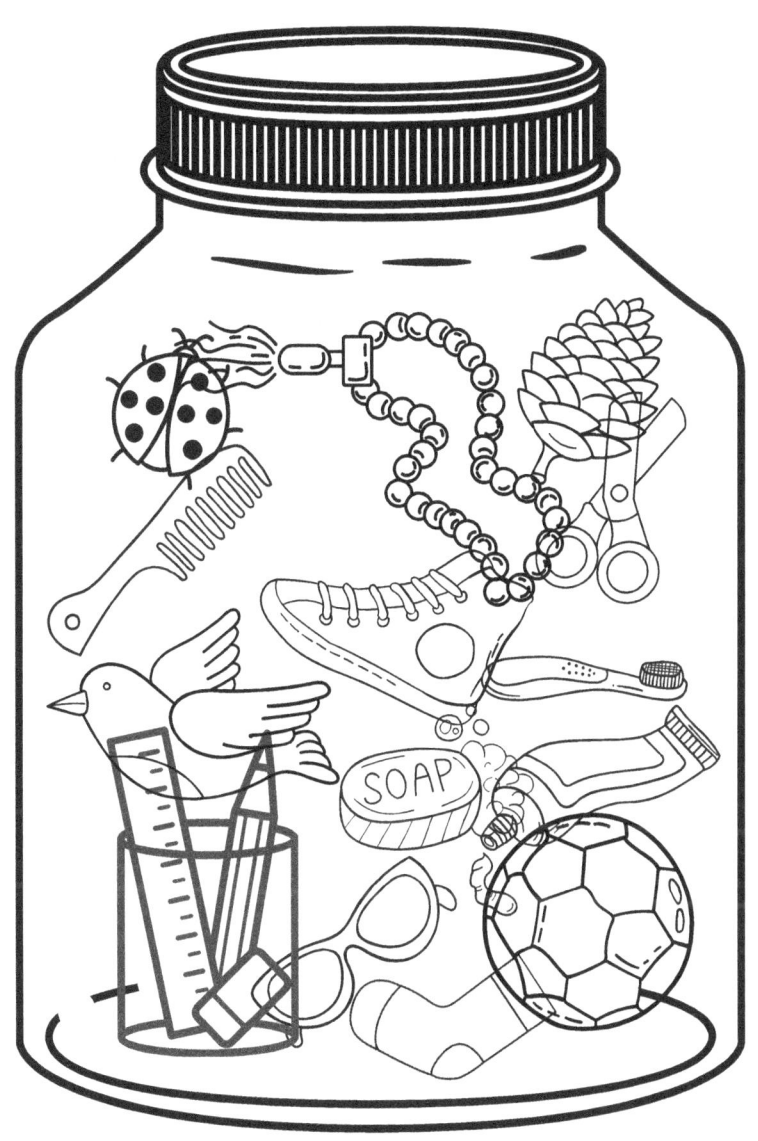

1. ....
2. ....
3. ....
4. ....
5. ....
6. ....
7. ....
8. ....
9. ....
10. ....
11. ....
12. ....
13. ....
14. ....

Reflection
ON MY MONTH

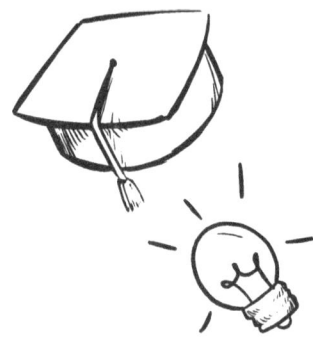

IMPORTANT *Goals* I ACHIEVED:

***High* POINTS:**

***Low* POINTS:**

MY *Favourite* THINGS:
- MUSIC ARTIST:
- MUSIC GENRE:
- LOCATION:
- FOOD:
- DRINK:
- SUBJECT:
- ACTIVITY:
- MOVIE:
- TV SHOW:
- EVENT:
- PURCHASE:
- TREAT:

THINGS I *Learnt*:

I AM *Grateful* FOR:

Images* OR SYMBOLS:

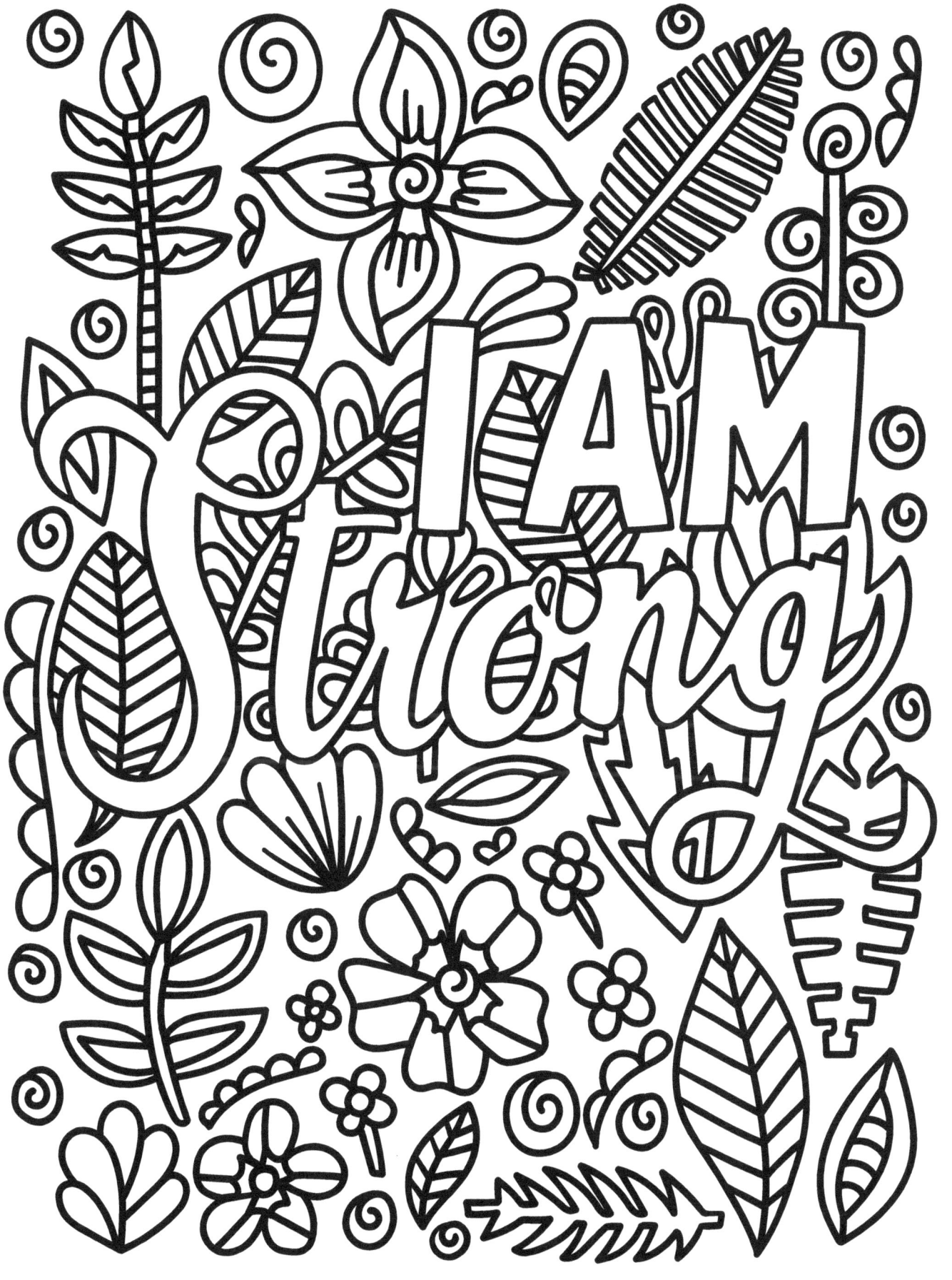

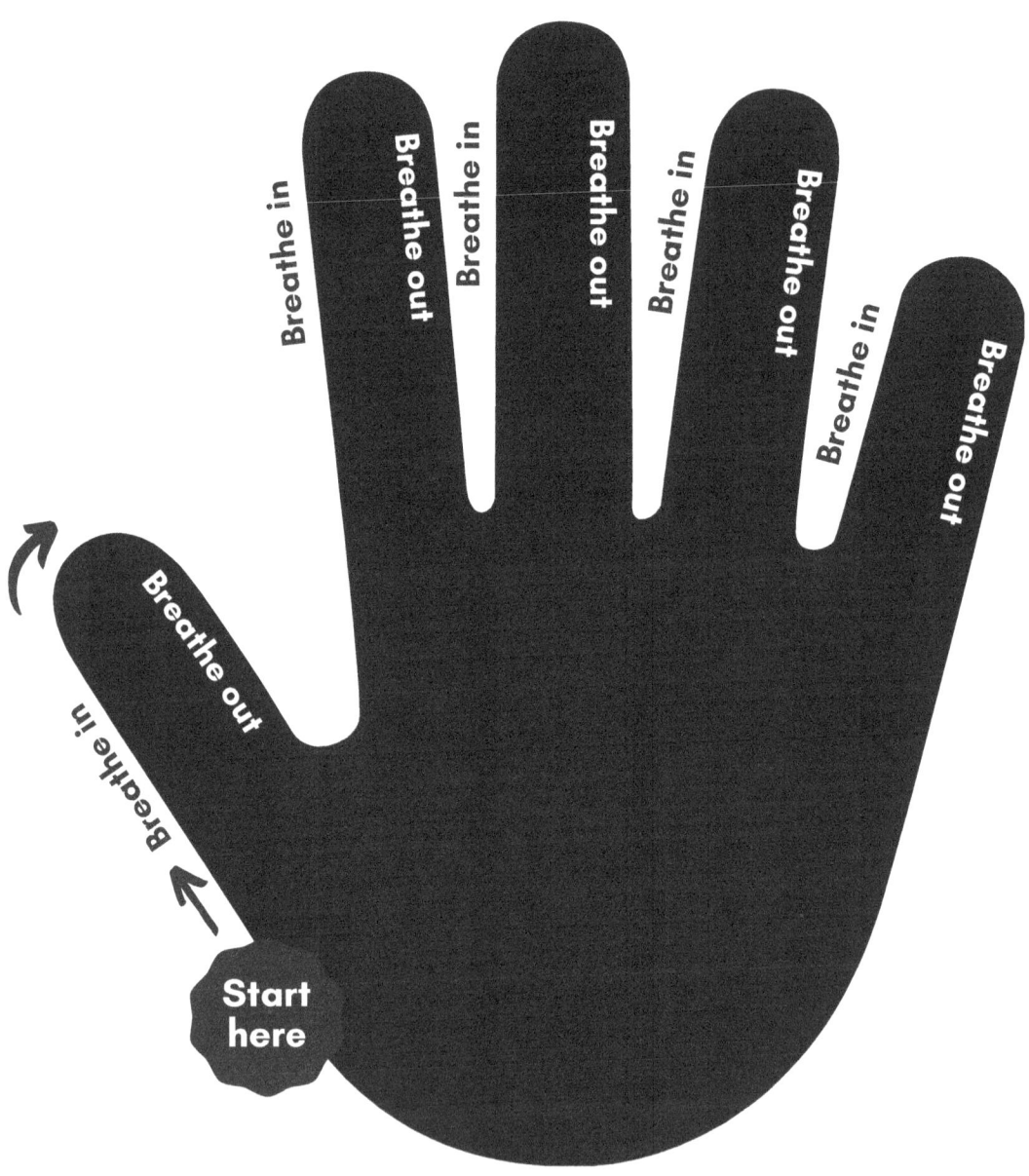

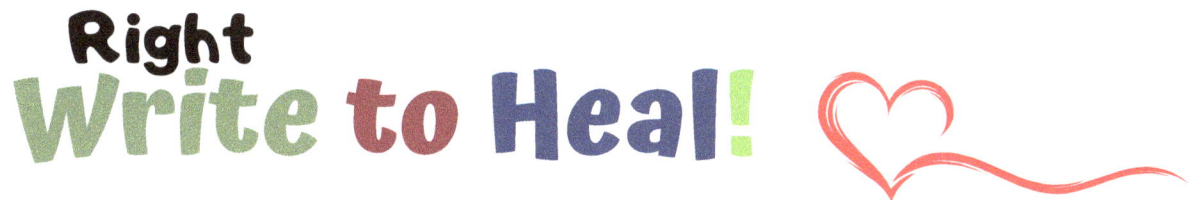

Right Write to Heal!

Writing about yourself in a poem is like giving your heart a hug.

When you talk about how strong, beautiful, or kind you are, it reminds you of all the good things inside. This can make you feel happy, confident, and proud of yourself! It's like magic—you're using words to heal yourself and feel better!

Let's write a poem that celebrates YOU and all the amazing things that make you strong and beautiful! You can choose between a haiku or an acrostic poem.

HERE'S HOW THEY WORK:

1. HAIKU

A haiku is a type of poem that has just 3 lines. Each line has a certain number of syllables:
- Line 1: 5 syllables
- Line 2: 7 syllables
- Line 3: 5 syllables

Haikus are usually short but powerful! They can be about anything—like your strength, your beauty, or what makes you special.

<u>Example of a Haiku:</u>
> I am full of light (5 syllables)
> My heart grows like a bright sun (7 syllables)
> Strong and proud, that's me! (5 syllables)

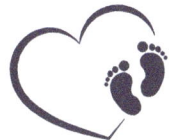

2. ACROSTIC POEM

An acrostic poem is where each line starts with a letter from a word. The word can be something you want to celebrate about yourself, like your name or a word like "STRONG" or "BRAVE."

For example, if your word is "BRAVE," you write a line starting with each letter:

Example of an Acrostic Poem for "BRAVE":
> **B**eaming with courage,
> **R**unning toward my dreams,
> **A**lways true to myself,
> **V**ictorious in every challenge,
> **E**very day, I grow stronger.

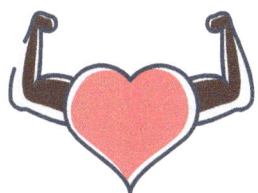

Right Write to Heal!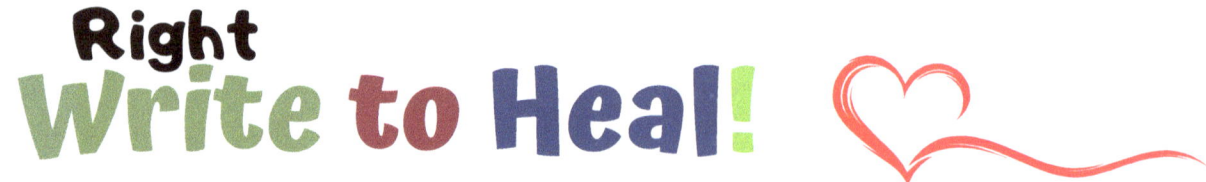

Your turn to write a poem that celebrates YOU and all the amazing things that make you strong and beautiful! You can choose between a haiku or an acrostic poem.

1. Choose your type of poem:
   a. haiku or
   b. acrostic
2. Pick your theme: Think about your strength, beauty, or anything that makes you feel proud of who you are.
3. Start writing: Follow the pattern for the haiku or acrostic, and let your words celebrate YOU!

You're going to create something special that shows the world just how amazing you are!

Mindful Coloring

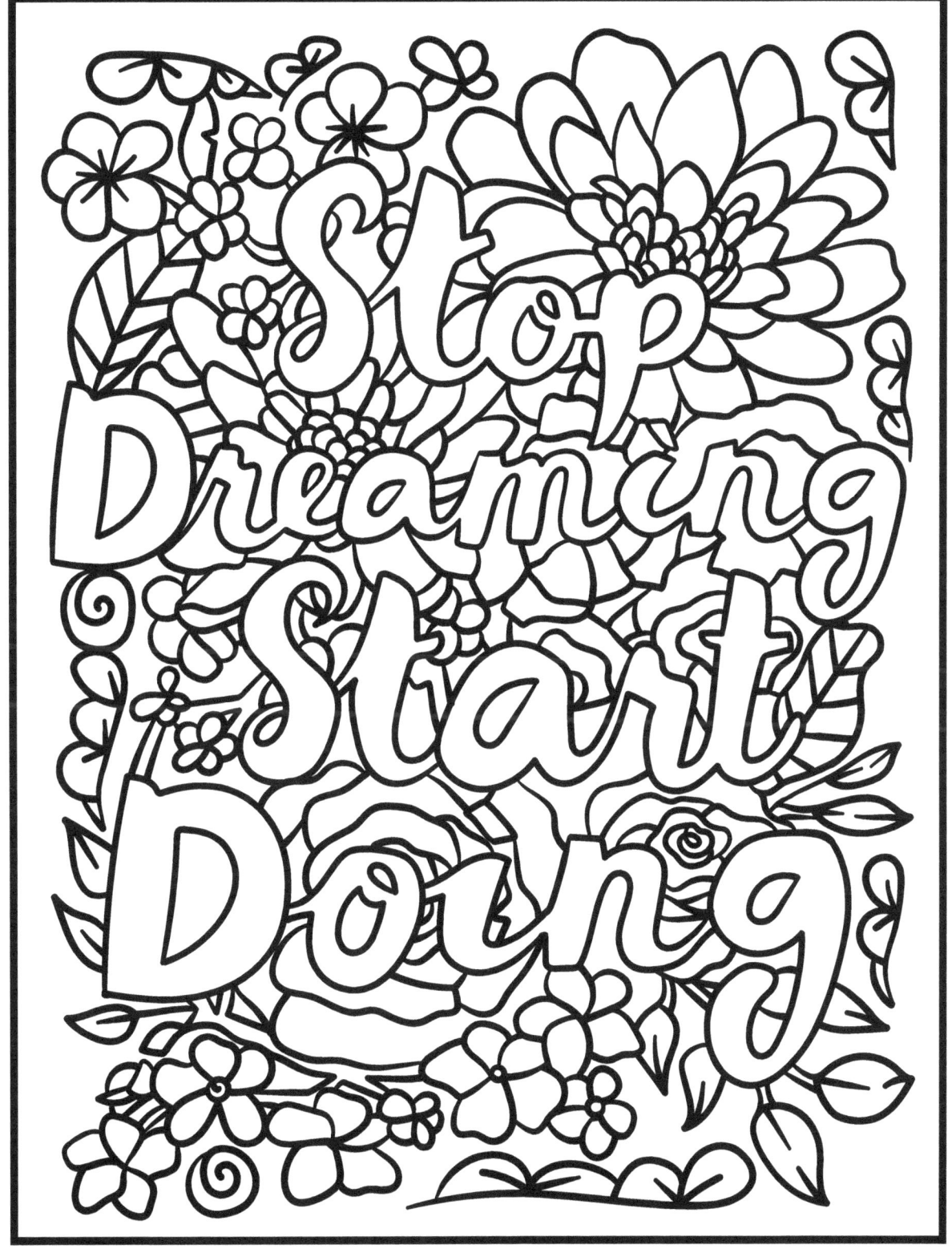

Today's dream record date: _____

_____
_____
_____
_____
_____
_____
_____
_____
_____
_____
_____
_____
_____
_____
_____
_____
_____

Follow your dreams and don't give up!

START YOUR NEW DAY WITH MINDFULNESS

1. Sit straight on a chair or on the floor.
2. Keep the back and the shoulders relaxed.
3. Close your eyes.
4. Breathe mindfully for five minutes.
5. Breathe in for 3 seconds, hold your breath for 4 seconds, and breathe out for 5 seconds. As you inhale, you breathe in love, joy, and peace. As you exhale, you breathe out sadness, boredom, anger, and tiredness.

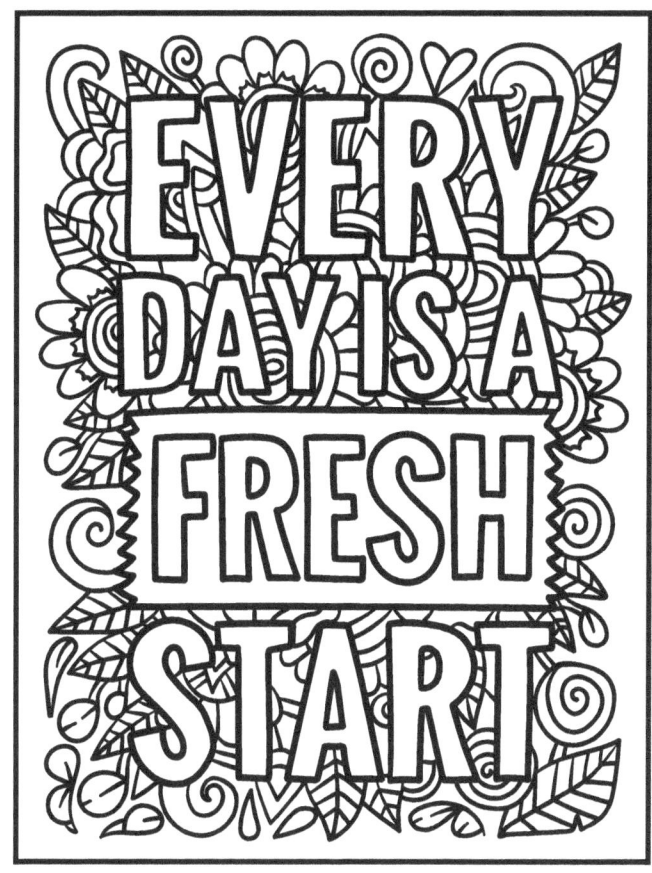

What emotions came up in your body and mind during this activity? Did your mind wander? What did you think about?

What does a fresh start look like for you?

PLANT LIFE!

WORD SEARCH – LEVEL 1

Find the words listed below and circle them.

L	S	P	O	L	L	E	N	Z	C	S	X
E	T	E	I	K	I	F	L	O	W	E	R
A	E	T	G	I	N	G	Y	A	M	I	L
V	M	A	I	S	F	R	O	N	P	L	S
E	M	L	G	K	R	O	Q	C	L	D	E
S	O	I	L	I	N	O	N	I	A	I	E
D	N	S	H	O	O	T	S	N	N	N	D
E	G	L	O	N	L	S	O	G	T	G	N
W	A	T	E	R	C	Y	C	L	I	F	E

- SEED
- WATER
- ROOTS
- POLLEN
- LEAVES
- PETAL
- STEM
- SHOOTS
- FLOWER
- PLANT
- LIFE
- SOIL

HARMONIOUS LIFE
tracker

Observe your mood, emotions and feelings.
Record all of your observations below.

month:

Emotions and feelings

	1	2	3	4	5	6	7	8	9	10	11	12	13	14	15	16	17	18	19	20	21	22	23	24	25	26	27	28	29	30	31
joy																															
calmness																															
happiness																															
love																															
gratitude																															
love																															
Excitement																															
Serenity																															
Peace																															
Appreciation																															
Bliss																															

Physical state

	1	2	3	4	5	6	7	8	9	10	11	12	13	14	15	16	17	18	19	20	21	22	23	24	25	26	27	28	29	30	31
sleep																															
physical activity																															
nutrition																															
body care																															
walk																															
happiness																															
creation																															
books																															

Reflections and goals

_____
_____
_____
_____
_____

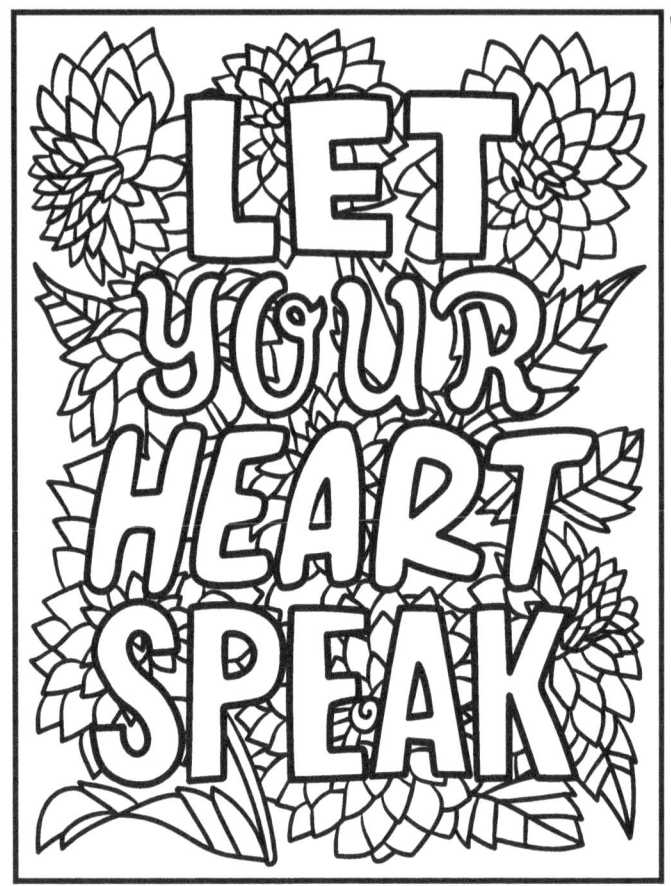

Write down five things that make you feel joyful.

Describe your happy place. What do you see, hear, feel, and smell in your happy place?

DRAW YOURSELF AS A SUPERHERO HERE

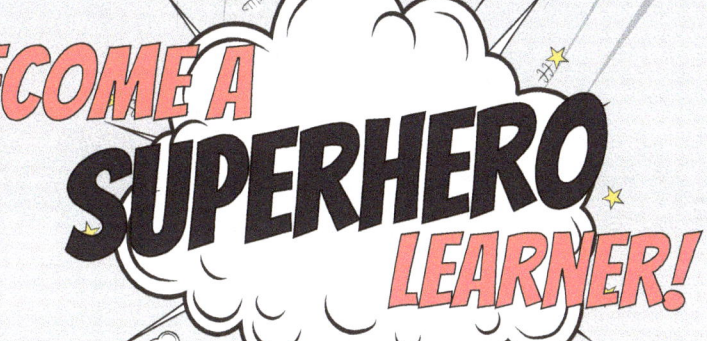
BECOME A SUPERHERO LEARNER!

WHAT ARE YOUR SUPERPOWERS?

YOUR SUPERHERO NAME

HOW WILL YOU OVERCOME THIS?

WHAT IS YOUR KRYPTONITE?

Name: Date:

MY SUPER STRENGTHS

Directions: Fill in the shapes with words that describe your strengths and what you like about yourself.

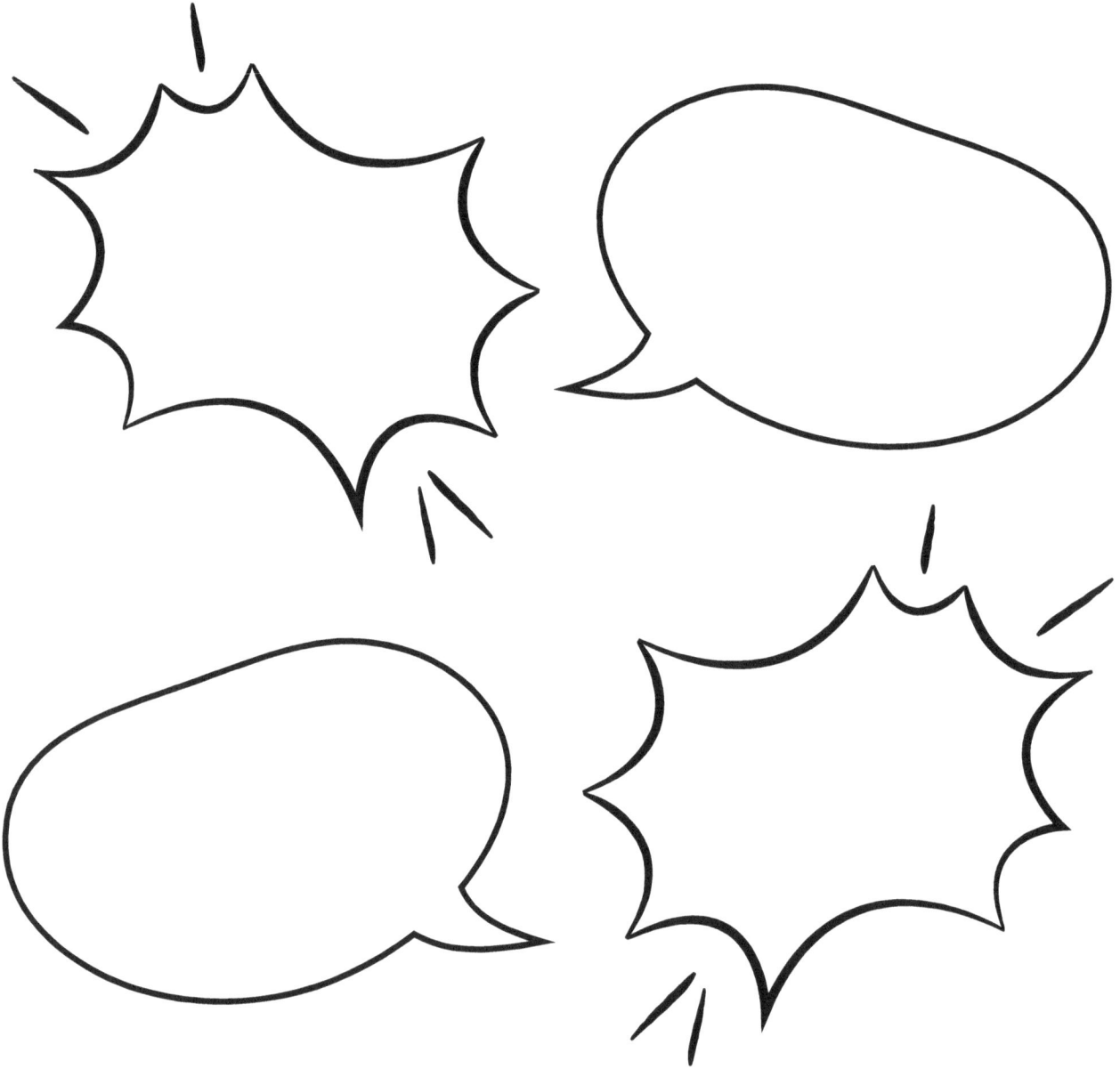

Ready to create your own superhero story?

Follow these steps to make an awesome adventure where the superpowers are self-love, self-awareness, and adventures in creation!

1. CREATE YOUR SUPERHERO
- Name: What's your superhero's name? It could be something cool like "Captain Confidence" or "Mindful Marvel"!
- Powers:
  - Self-Love: Your superhero loves who they are, inside and out. How do they show their self-love? Maybe they cheer themselves up when they're feeling down!
  - Self-Awareness: They always know what they're feeling and thinking. How does your hero use this power to stay calm or help others?
  - Adventures in Creation: This hero loves to make new things—maybe they create worlds, art, or new ideas! What awesome thing will your hero create to help save the day?

2. CHOOSE A PROBLEM
Every superhero story needs a problem to solve! Think of a challenge for your hero:
- Maybe there's a town that's feeling sad or people who are scared to be themselves.
- Or maybe the world is losing its color, and your superhero has to create beauty and joy again.

3. WRITE ABOUT THE ADVENTURE
Now, let your superhero save the day! Here are some things to include:
- How does your superhero use their powers? Does their self-love make them brave? Does their self-awareness help them make good decisions?
- What do they create during the adventure? Maybe they draw something magical or come up with a new idea to solve the problem.
- Who do they help along the way? Are there other characters who need a little help loving themselves or creating something special?

4. THE BIG MOMENT
- How does your hero solve the problem? Do they help others learn to love themselves too? Do they create something beautiful that changes the world? Write about how your superhero uses all their powers to make everything better!

5. THE ENDING
- How does your superhero feel at the end of the story? What have they learned from their adventure? Maybe they've helped others become more confident or more creative.

Now go ahead and start writing your amazing superhero adventure! Remember, your hero's greatest powers come from inside them, and they can use them to make the world a better.

WE HEAL IN COMMUNITY

Who are the people I feel I can turn to when I'm feeling overwhelmed, sad, or in need of support?

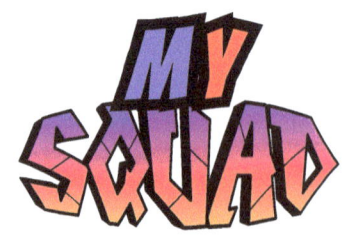

Reflect on the power of community and how the presence of others enhances your growth and healing.

Who are the people with whom I find joy, peace, and love when I am with them?

What qualities do I appreciate most in the people I consider part of my community?

How can I continue to nurture and strengthen these relationships so that I feel more supported in my healing?

What are ways you can or do show appreciation for the people in your life who hold space for your well-being?

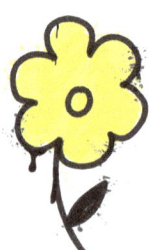

Word Search

Create your own word Search using the names of your family.

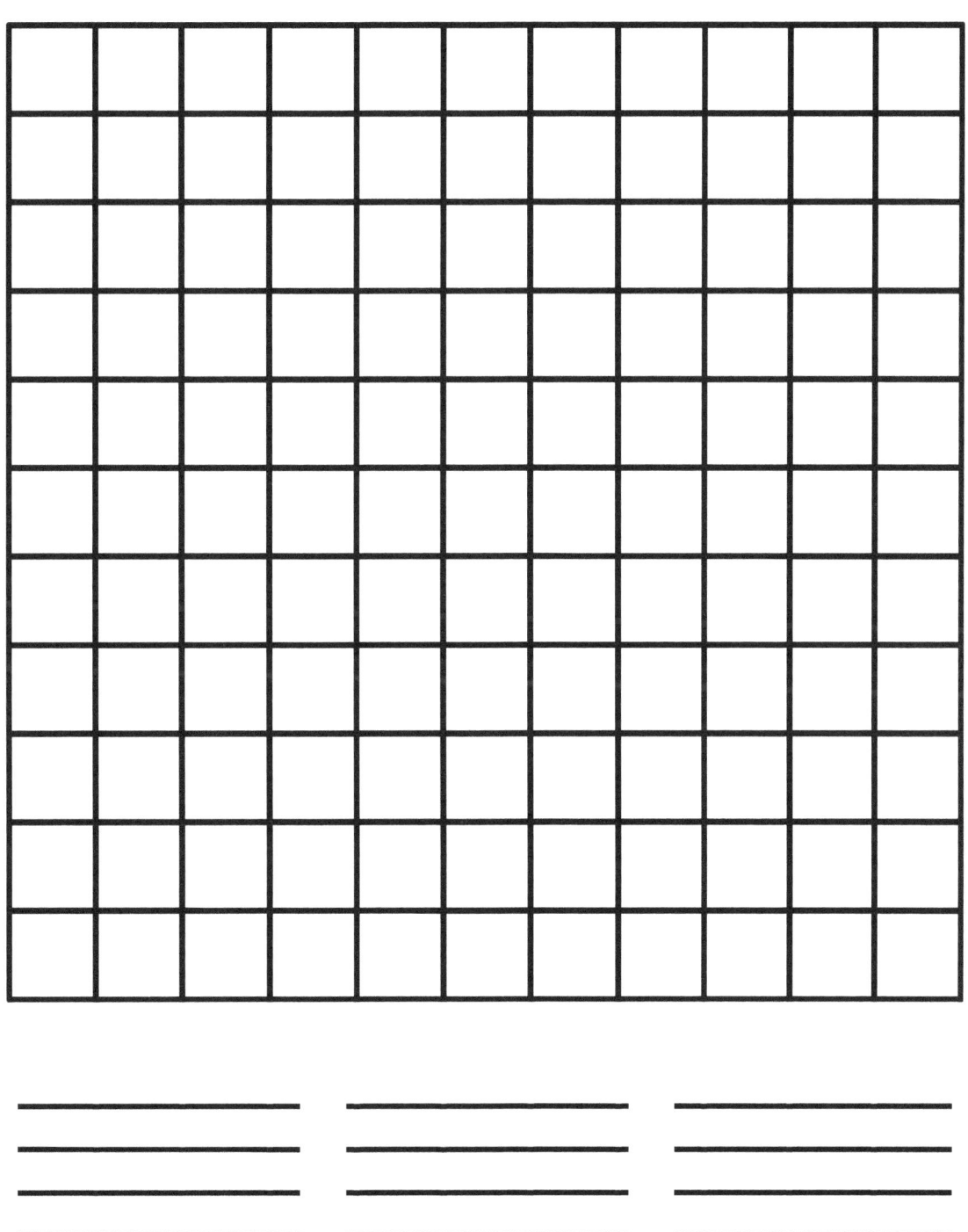

Create a "Joy List" of music that heals the heart and soul

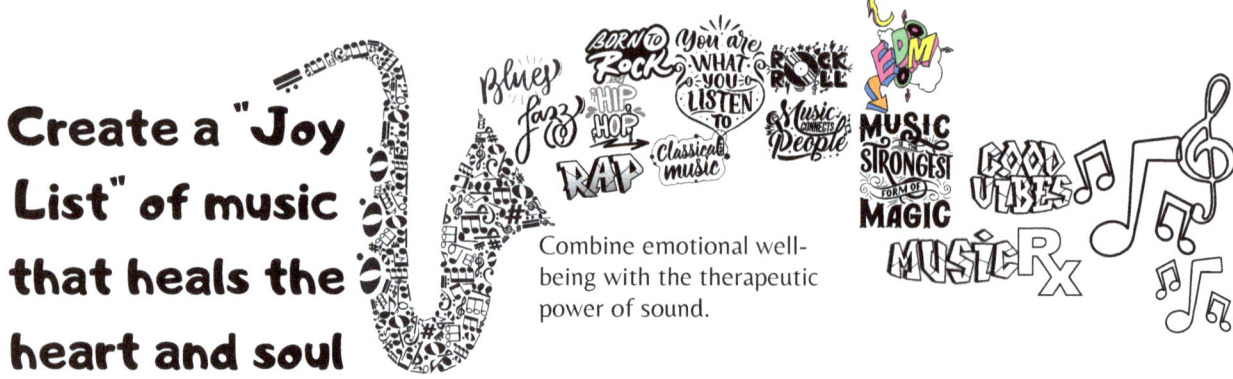

Combine emotional well-being with the therapeutic power of sound.

1. Reflect on Your Emotional Needs
- Begin by asking yourself: What kind of music uplifts or soothes me? What songs or sounds make me feel safe, loved, or grounded?
- Identify how different songs or genres affect your mood. For instance, some music may make you feel energized, while others might provide calmness or clarity.

2. Choose Heart-Centered Music
- Healing frequencies: Consider music that incorporates healing frequencies such as 432Hz or 528Hz, which are known to calm the nervous system.
- Lyrics with meaning: Include songs that resonate with themes of hope, love, and resilience. The lyrics should remind you of your inner strength and beauty, lifting your spirits even when you feel down.
- Genres to explore: Classical, instrumental, soul, gospel, world music, and nature sounds can be profoundly soothing.

3. Gather Songs That Spark Joy and Healing
- Think of songs that bring back happy memories, remind you of loved ones, or simply make you smile. These songs will be the core of your Joy List.
- Pay attention to both the melody and lyrics. Songs with slow rhythms or uplifting melodies can have a soothing effect on the body and mind.
- Examples of mood-boosting songs might include:
  - Calming instrumental pieces
  - Soulful ballads that resonate with your emotions
  - Songs with positive, uplifting lyrics

4. Create Playlists for Different Moods
- Soothing: Include soft, ambient tracks that help you slow down and reconnect with yourself. This can be used during moments of anxiety or nervous system overload.
- Uplifting: Songs that energize you when feeling low, bringing lightness and joy to your heart.
- Grounding: Music with nature sounds or repetitive, calming rhythms to help you feel rooted and safe.

5. Use the Music for Emotional Regulation
- Mindful listening: When feeling sad or overwhelmed, find a quiet space and play your Joy List. Close your eyes, breathe deeply, and allow yourself to fully experience the music. Let it wash over you, calming your mind and body.
- Deep breathing: Synchronize your breath with the music. Inhale deeply through your nose for a count of 4, hold for 4, and exhale through your mouth for a count of 6 or 8. This activates the parasympathetic nervous system, which aids in calming the body.
- Movement: If it feels right, sway, stretch, or dance to the music. Allow the music to guide your movements as a way to release tension and reconnect with joy.
- Repeat affirmations: While listening, try repeating self-soothing affirmations that align with the music's message. For example, "I am loved," "I am whole," or "I trust in my ability to heal."

6. Regular Practice
- Make listening to your Joy List a regular part of your self-care routine. Play it when you wake up, during a mindfulness practice, or whenever you need a mental and emotional reset.

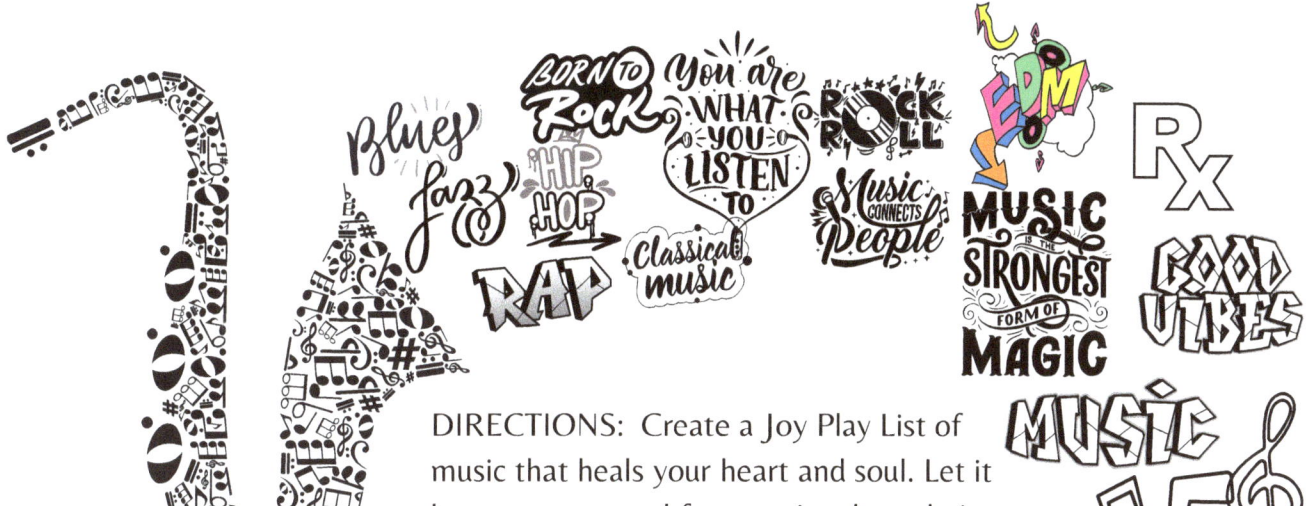

DIRECTIONS: Create a Joy Play List of music that heals your heart and soul. Let it be your go-to tool for emotional regulation. May it remind you that even in moments of sadness, you have the power to uplift and soothe your spirit.

Song Title:	Artist/Composer:	How It Heals Me: (Example: "Reminds me of peaceful moments, calms my anxiety, uplifts my mood")

MY JOY PLAYLIST

LETTER
to myself

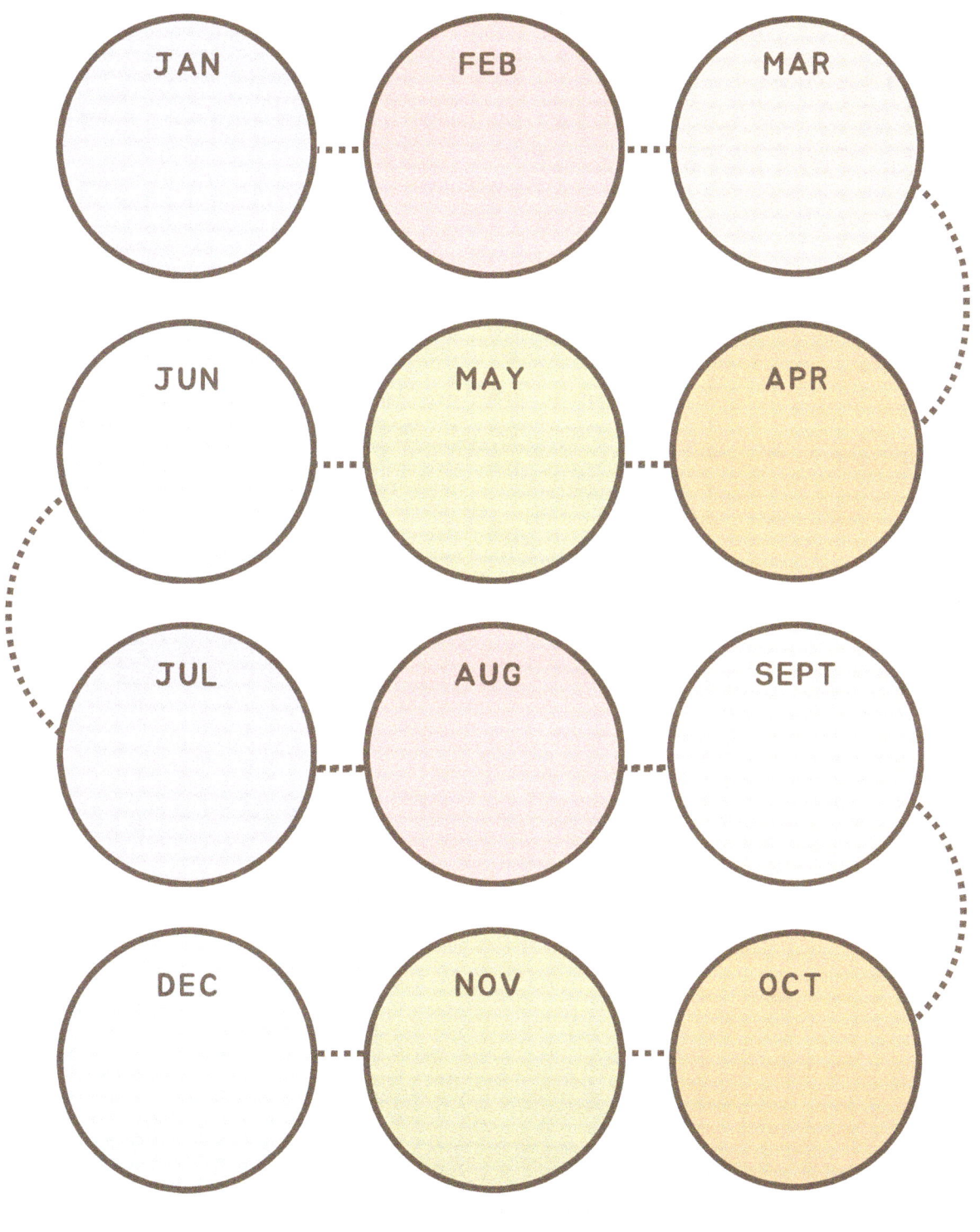

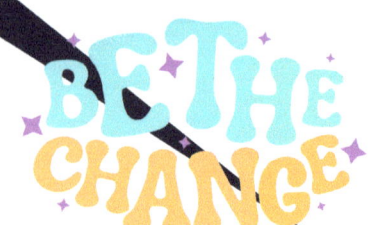

MONTHLY PLANNER

MONDAY	TUESDAY	WEDNESDAY	THURSDAY	FRIDAY	SATURDAY

NOTES:

....

....

....

....

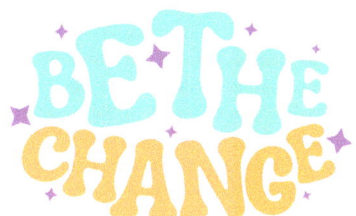

MONTHLY PLANNER

MONDAY	TUESDAY	WEDNESDAY	THURSDAY	FRIDAY	SATURDAY

NOTES:

....

....

....

....

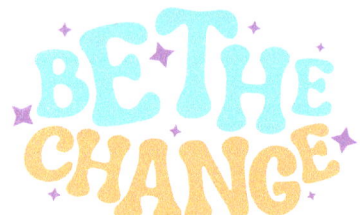

MONTHLY PLANNER

MONDAY	TUESDAY	WEDNESDAY	THURSDAY	FRIDAY	SATURDAY

NOTES:

....

....

....

....

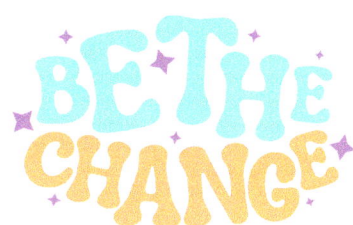

MONTHLY PLANNER

MONDAY	TUESDAY	WEDNESDAY	THURSDAY	FRIDAY	SATURDAY

NOTES:

....

....

....

....

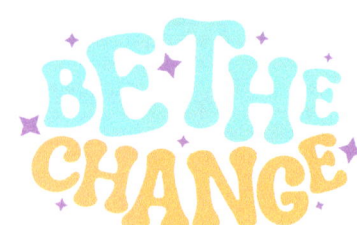

MONTHLY PLANNER

MONDAY	TUESDAY	WEDNESDAY	THURSDAY	FRIDAY	SATURDAY

NOTES:

....

....

....

....

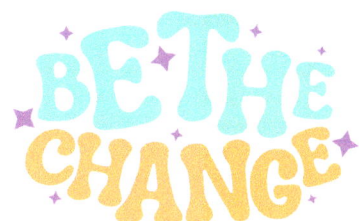

MONTHLY PLANNER

MONDAY	TUESDAY	WEDNESDAY	THURSDAY	FRIDAY	SATURDAY

NOTES:

....

....

....

....

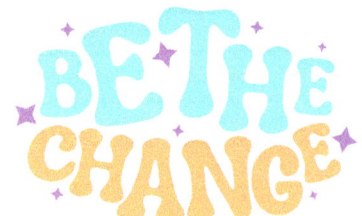

MONTHLY PLANNER

MONDAY	TUESDAY	WEDNESDAY	THURSDAY	FRIDAY	SATURDAY

NOTES:

....
....
....
....

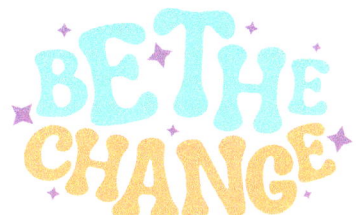

MONTHLY PLANNER

MONDAY	TUESDAY	WEDNESDAY	THURSDAY	FRIDAY	SATURDAY

NOTES:

....

....

....

....

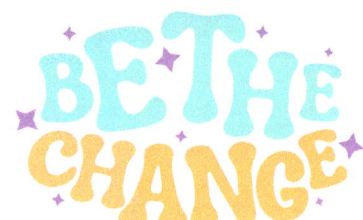

MONTHLY PLANNER

MONDAY	TUESDAY	WEDNESDAY	THURSDAY	FRIDAY	SATURDAY

NOTES:

....

....

....

....

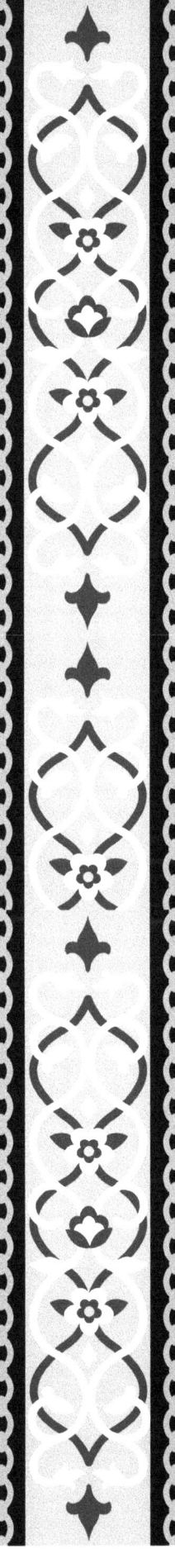

SEVEN QUALITIES LOVED by THE DIVINE ONE......

1- TAWBAH (Repentance) "For Allah Loves those who turn to Him Constantly (in repentance)" (Surat Al- Baqarah 2:222)

2- TAQWA (Piety) "For Allah Loves the righteous (the pious)" (Surat Al- Tawabah 9:4)

3- TAHARAH (Purification) Allah Loves those who keep themselves pure and clean " (Surah Al- Baqarah 2:222)

4- IHSAN (Goodness and perfection) "For Allah Loves those who do good ",(Surah Al Imran 3:134)

5- TAWWAKAL (Trust in Allah) For Allah Loves those who put their trust (in Him) Surah Al Imran 3:159)

6- ADL (Justice) For Allah Loves those who judge in equity " (Surah Al Ma'idah 5:42)

7- SABR (Patience) And Allah Loves those who are firm and steadfast (As- Sabinn) (the patient) (Surah Al Imran 3:146).

About the author

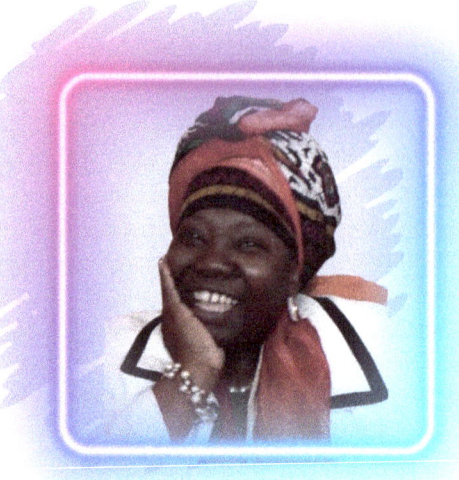

Qur'an Shakir, affectionately called Madame Q, has written this book as a companion and friend to those that need a safe space to unpack thoughts and emotions. Madame Q believes that not enough support is given to those struggling emotionally. She is a distinguished advocate for children, marriage, empowered women, griot (keeper of the history and traditions), and is recognized across the U.S. for her championship work as a master teacher, Jegna, and an award-winning educator. Madame Q said her greatest joy and accomplishment is being a graduate of the University of the Creator Advanced Practice Professional Umm --a mom and a grandmother.

ISBN: 97989896332-4-1

www.ingramcontent.com/pod-product-compliance
Lightning Source LLC
Chambersburg PA
CBHW042357030426
42337CB00030B/5134